Sleep and Performance

Editors

RACHEL R. MARKWALD
ANNE GERMAIN

SLEEP MEDICINE CLINICS

www.sleep.theclinics.com

Consulting Editor
TEOFILO LEE-CHIONG Jr

March 2020 • Volume 15 • Number 1

ELSEVIER

1600 John F. Kennedy Boulevard ● Suite 1800 ● Philadelphia, Pennsylvania, 19103-2899

http://www.theclinics.com

SLEEP MEDICINE CLINICS Volume 15, Number 1
March 2020, ISSN 1556-407X, ISBN-13: 978-0-323-68360-9

Editor: Colleen Dietzler
Developmental Editor: Donald Mumford

Sleep Medicine Clinics (ISSN 1556-407X) is published quarterly by Elsevier Inc., 360 Park Avenue South, New York, NY 10010-1710. Months of issue are March, June, September and December. Business and Editorial Offices: 1600 John F. Kennedy Blvd., Ste. 1800, Philadelphia, PA 19103-2899. Customer Service Office: 3251 Riverport Lane, Maryland Heights, MO 63043. Periodicals postage paid at New York, NY and additional mailing offices. Subscription prices are $218.00 per year (US individuals), $100.00 (US and Canadian students), $518.00 (US institutions), $264.00 (Canadian individuals), $252.00 (international individuals) $135.00 (International students), $587.00 (Canadian and International institutions). Foreign air speed delivery is included in all *Clinics* subscription prices. All prices are subject to change without notice. **POSTMASTER:** Send change of address to *Sleep Medicine Clinics*, Elsevier Health Sciences Division, Subscription Customer Service, 3251 Riverport Lane, Maryland Heights, MO 63043. Customer Service: **Tel: 1-800-654-2452 (U.S. and Canada); 314-447-8871 (outside U.S. and Canada). Fax: 314-447-8029. E-mail: journalscustomerservice-usa@elsevier.com (for print support); journalsonline-support-usa@elsevier.com (for online support).**

Reprints. For copies of 100 or more of articles in this publication, please contact the Commercial Reprints Department, Elsevier Inc., 360 Park Avenue South, New York, NY 10010-1710. Tel.: 212-633-3874; Fax: 212-633-3820; E-mail: reprints@elsevier.com.

Sleep Medicine Clinics is covered in *MEDLINE/PubMed (Index Medicus)*.

SLEEP MEDICINE CLINICS

FORTHCOMING ISSUES

June 2020
Essentials of Sleep Medicine for the Primary Care Provider
Teofilo Lee-Chong, *Editor*

September 2020
Telehealth in Sleep Medicine
Jean Louis Pépin and Dennis Hwang, *Editors*

December 2020
Noninvasive Ventilation and Sleep Medicine
Amen Sergew and Lisa Wolfe, *Editors*

RECENT ISSUES

December 2019
Sleep And Driving
Walter T. McNicholas, *Editor*

September 2019
Precision Sleep Medicine
Susheel P. Patil, *Editor*

June 2019
Cognitive Behavioral Therapies for Insomnia
Jason C. Ong, *Editor*

SERIES OF RELATED INTEREST

Clinics in Chest Medicine
Available at: https://www.chestmed.theclinics.com/

THE CLINICS ARE AVAILABLE ONLINE!
Access your subscription at:
www.theclinics.com

Contributors

CONSULTING EDITOR

TEOFILO LEE-CHIONG Jr, MD
Professor of Medicine, National Jewish Health,
University of Colorado Denver, Denver,
Colorado, USA; Chief Medical Liaison, Philips
Respironics, Pennsylvania, USA

EDITORS

RACHEL R. MARKWALD, PhD
Director, Sleep and Fatigue Research
Laboratory, Warfighter Performance
Department, Naval Health Research Center,
San Diego, California, USA

ANNE GERMAIN, PhD
Professor of Psychiatry, University of
Pittsburgh School of Medicine; CEO, Rehat
LLC (dba NOCTEM), Pittsburgh, Pennsylvania,
USA

AUTHORS

FIONA C. BAKER, PhD
Center for Health Sciences, SRI International,
Menlo Park, California, USA; Brain Function
Research Group, School of Physiology,
University of the Witwatersrand,
Johannesburg, South Africa

ALLISON BRAGER, PhD
Human Performance Operations and
Education Recruiting Outreach Company,
United States Army Recruiting Command, Fort
Knox, Kentucky, USA

MATTHEW S. BROCK, MD
Department of Sleep Medicine, Wilford Hall
Ambulatory Surgical Center, San Antonio,
Texas, USA

JANEESE A. BROWNLOW, PhD
Department of Psychology, College of Health &
Behavioral Sciences, Delaware State
University, Dover, Delaware, USA; Department
of Psychiatry, Perelman School of Medicine,
University of Pennsylvania, Philadelphia,
Pennsylvania, USA

NICOLA CELLINI, PhD
Department of General Psychology,
Department of Biomedical Sciences, Padova
Neuroscience Center, Human Inspired
Technology Center, University of Padua,
Padua, Italy

JONATHAN CHAREST
PhD Candidate, Department of Psychology,
Université Laval, Quebec City, Quebec,
Canada; Behavioral Sleep Medicine Specialist,
Centre for Sleep and Human Performance,
Calgary, Alberta, Canada

JACOB COLLEN, MD
Uniformed Services University of the Health
Sciences, Bethesda, Maryland, USA

CHRISTOPHER CONNABOY, PhD
Department of Sports Medicine and Nutrition,
University of Pittsburgh, Pittsburgh,
Pennsylvania, USA

MASSIMILIANO de ZAMBOTTI, PhD
Center for Health Sciences, SRI International,
Menlo Park, California, USA

SHAWN R. EAGLE, PhD, ATC, CSCS
Rooney Sports Medicine Concussion Program, Department of Orthopaedic Surgery, University of Pittsburgh Medical Center, University of Pittsburgh School of Medicine, Pittsburgh, Pennsylvania, USA

FABIO FERRARELLI, MD, PhD
Department of Psychiatry, University of Pittsburgh School of Medicine, Pittsburgh, Pennsylvania, USA

PHILIP R. GEHRMAN, PhD, CBSM
Department of Psychiatry, Perelman School of Medicine, University of Pennsylvania, Mental Illness Research, Education, and Clinical Center, Corporal Michael J. Crescenz VA Medical Center, Philadelphia, Pennsylvania, USA

MICHAEL A. GRANDNER, PhD, MTR
Associate Professor, Department of Psychiatry, The University of Arizona, Tucson, Arizona, USA

TONY S. HAN, MD
Assistant Professor of Medicine, Uniformed Services University, Pulmonary Medicine Department, Naval Medical Center San Diego, San Diego, California, USA

CALEB D. JOHNSON, PhD
Department of Physical Medicine and Rehabilitation, Harvard Medical School, Cambridge, Massachusetts, USA

ALICE D. LAGOY, MS
Department of Sports Medicine and Nutrition, University of Pittsburgh, Department of Psychiatry, University of Pittsburgh School of Medicine, Pittsburgh, Pennsylvania, USA

MATTHEW LoPRESTI, PhD
US Army Medical Research Directorate-West, Walter Reed Army Institute of Research, USA

RONEIL G. MALKANI, MD, MS
Assistant Professor of Neurology, Division of Sleep Medicine, Department of Neurology, Center for Circadian and Sleep Medicine,

Northwestern University Feinberg School of Medicine, Chicago, Illinois, USA

LUCA MENGHINI, MS
Department of General Psychology, University of Padua, Padua, Italy

KATHERINE E. MILLER, PhD
Mental Illness Research, Education, and Clinical Center, Corporal Michael J. Crescenz VA Medical Center, Philadelphia, Pennsylvania, USA

BRIAN A. MOORE, PhD
The University of Texas Health Science Center at San Antonio, The University of Texas at San Antonio, San Antonio, Texas, USA

VINCENT MYSLIWIEC, MD
The University of Texas Health Science Center at San Antonio, San Antonio, Texas, USA

J. ROXANNE PRICHARD, PhD
Professor of Psychology, University of St. Thomas, St Paul, Minnesota, USA

MICHELA SARLO, PhD
Department of General Psychology and Padova Neuroscience Center, University of Padua, Padua, Italy

GILBERT SEDA, MD, PhD
Associate Professor of Medicine, Uniformed Services University, Pulmonary Medicine Department, Naval Medical Center San Diego, San Diego, California, USA

AARON M. SINNOTT, MS, ATC
Department of Sports Medicine and Nutrition, University of Pittsburgh, Pittsburgh, Pennsylvania, USA

PHYLLIS C. ZEE, MD, PhD
Professor of Neurology, Division of Sleep Medicine, Department of Neurology, Center for Circadian and Sleep Medicine, Northwestern University Feinberg School of Medicine, Chicago, Illinois, USA

Contents

Preface: Waking Up to the Impacts of Sleep Health on Human Performance   xi

Rachel R. Markwald and Anne Germain

Sensors Capabilities, Performance, and Use of Consumer Sleep Technology   1

Massimiliano de Zambotti, Nicola Cellini, Luca Menghini, Michela Sarlo, and Fiona C. Baker

> Sleep is crucial for the proper functioning of bodily systems and for cognitive and emotional processing. Evidence indicates that sleep is vital for health, well-being, mood, and performance. Consumer sleep technologies (CSTs), such as multisensory wearable devices, have brought attention to sleep and there is growing interest in using CSTs in research and clinical applications. This article reviews how CSTs can process information about sleep, physiology, and environment. The growing number of sensors in wearable devices and the meaning of the data collected are reviewed. CSTs have the potential to provide opportunities to measure sleep and sleep-related physiology on a large scale.

You Snooze, You Win? An Ecological Dynamics Framework Approach to Understanding the Relationships Between Sleep and Sensorimotor Performance in Sport   31

Alice D. LaGoy, Fabio Ferrarelli, Aaron M. Sinnott, Shawn R. Eagle, Caleb D. Johnson, and Christopher Connaboy

> Sleep has a widespread impact across different domains of performance, including sensorimotor function. From an ecological dynamics perspective, sensorimotor function involves the continuous and dynamic coupling between perception and action. Sport performance relies on sensorimotor function as successful movement behaviors require accurate and efficient coupling between perceptions and actions. Compromised sleep impairs different aspects of sensorimotor performance, including perceptual attunement and motor execution. Changes in sensorimotor performance can be related to specific features of sleep, notably sleep spindles and slow waves. One unaddressed area of study is the extent to which specific sleep features contribute to overall sport-specific performance.

Sleep and Athletic Performance: Impacts on Physical Performance, Mental Performance, Injury Risk and Recovery, and Mental Health   41

Jonathan Charest and Michael A. Grandner

> Research has characterized the sleep of elite athletes and attempted to identify factors associated with athletic performance, cognition, health, and mental well-being. Sleep is a fundamental component of performance optimization among elite athletes, yet only recently embraced by sport organizations as an important part of training and recovery. Sleep plays a crucial role in physical and cognitive performance and is an important factor in reducing risk of injury. This article aims to highlight the prevalence of poor sleep, describe its impacts, and address the issue of sport culture surrounding healthy sleep.

Sleep Predicts Collegiate Academic Performance: Implications for Equity in Student Retention and Success   59

J. Roxanne Prichard

> College students show high levels of insufficient sleep, excessive daytime sleepiness, sleep schedule irregularity, poor sleep quality, and inadequate sleep hygiene.

This article describes the evidence linking poor sleep with impaired academic performance; discusses mediating environmental, behavioral, and demographic factors that correlate with sleep; and highlights examples of successful health promotion initiatives on college campuses. Given that students who are traditionally minoritized on college campuses tend to have worse sleep, improving sleep health emerges as an important issue for retention, equity, and inclusion.

Insomnia and Cognitive Performance   71

Janeese A. Brownlow, Katherine E. Miller, and Philip R. Gehrman

Insomnia is the most common sleep problem, affecting between 30% and 50% in the general adult population. Insomnia is characterized by difficulty initiating and maintaining sleep, along with dissatisfaction with sleep quality or quantity. Insomnia complaints are linked to clinically significant distress or impairment in key areas of functioning, especially daytime cognitive performance. Cognitive impairments related to insomnia are subtle, and may represent distinct differences from those seen in other sleep disorders. This article updates and summarizes the recent literature investigating cognitive impairments in individuals with insomnia, and identifies the cognitive domains of functioning that are consistently impaired.

Effect of Obstructive Sleep Apnea on Neurocognitive Performance   77

Gilbert Seda and Tony S. Han

This article reviews the effects of obstructive sleep apnea on neurocognitive performance, proposed mechanisms of cognitive impairment, and the effects of continuous positive airway pressure on performance. Obstructive sleep apnea can affect several domains of neurocognitive performance to include attention and vigilance, memory and learning, psychomotor function, emotional regulation, and executive function. Proposed mechanisms include intermittent hypoxemia, sleep deprivation and fragmentation, hypercapnia, and disruption of the hypothalamic-pituitary-adrenal-axis. Continuous positive airway pressure can improve cognitive defects associated with obstructive sleep apnea. More data are needed to determine whether other therapies improve cognitive function.

Posttraumatic Stress Disorder, Traumatic Brain Injury, Sleep, and Performance in Military Personnel   87

Brian A. Moore, Matthew S. Brock, Allison Brager, Jacob Collen, Matthew LoPresti, and Vincent Mysliwiec

Sleep disturbances, posttraumatic stress disorder, and traumatic brain injury are highly prevalent in military personnel and veterans. These disorders can negatively impact military performance. Although literature evaluating how posttraumatic stress disorder and traumatic brain injury directly impact military performance is limited, there is evidence supporting that these disorders negatively impact cognitive and social functioning. What is not clear is if impaired performance results from these entities individually, or a combination of each. Further research using standardized evaluations for the clinical disorders and metrics of military performance is required to assess the overall performance decrements related to these disorders.

Brain Stimulation for Improving Sleep and Memory   101

Roneil G. Malkani and Phyllis C. Zee

Given the critical role of sleep, particularly sleep slow oscillations, sleep spindles, and hippocampal sharp wave ripples, in memory consolidation, sleep enhancement represents a key opportunity to improve cognitive performance. Techniques such as transcranial electrical and magnetic stimulation and acoustic stimulation can enhance slow oscillations and sleep spindles and potentially improve memory. Targeted memory reactivation in sleep may enhance or stabilize memory consolidation. Each technique has technical considerations that may limit its broader clinical application. Therefore, neurostimulation to enhance sleep quality, in particular sleep slow oscillations, has the potential for improving sleep-related memory consolidation in healthy and clinical populations.

Preface

Waking Up to the Impacts of Sleep Health on Human Performance

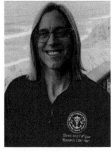 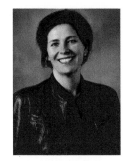

Rachel R. Markwald, PhD   Anne Germain, PhD

Editors

Several decades of research conducted in controlled laboratory settings have illuminated the impact of inadequate sleep quality and/or quantity on neurocognitive performance as well as psychological and physical fitness, readiness, and health. While the magnitude of these effects varies with individual and contextual differences, and across constructs and domains of interest, the findings overwhelmingly indicate a deleterious effect of inadequate sleep on human performance and health. Moving from laboratory assessments into clinical, competitive athletics, and occupational settings, research studies are demonstrating that inadequate sleep has real-world implications on sport and academic performance, recovery from psychological and physical injury/illness, and occupational health and safety. Growing evidence demonstrates that targeting the reestablishment of restorative, sufficient, and consolidated sleep through evidence-based prevention strategies and treatments is accompanied with improvements in performance and clinical outcomes. Novel measurement methods and intervention approaches can play a significant role in translating basic and clinical research findings into effective means of enhancing performance and health across populations. The following articles provide a review of the current research available within these topic areas.

Furthermore, because sleep measurement has expanded beyond the laboratory and clinic into the public health domain, we open this issue with an extensive review on the use and limitations of consumer sleep tracking devices for clinical and human performance research applications. Last, there have been recent advances in the development of neurostimulation technologies for enhancing sleep and performance, and this issue will close with a review on the current research available on these emerging approaches.

Rachel R. Markwald, PhD
Sleep and Fatigue Research Laboratory
Warfighter Performance Department
Naval Health Research Center
140 Sylvester Road
San Diego, CA 92101, USA

Anne Germain, PhD
University of Pittsburgh
School of Medicine
NOCTEM
218 Oakland Avenue
Pittsburgh, PA 15213, USA

E-mail addresses:
Rachel.r.markwald.civ@mail.mil (R.R. Markwald)
germax@upmc.edu (A. Germain)

Sleep Med Clin 15 (2020) xi
https://doi.org/10.1016/j.jsmc.2020.01.001
1556-407X/20/© 2020 Published by Elsevier Inc.

Sensors Capabilities, Performance, and Use of Consumer Sleep Technology

Massimiliano de Zambotti, PhD[a],*, Nicola Cellini, PhD[b,c,d,e], Luca Menghini, MS[b], Michela Sarlo, PhD[b,d], Fiona C. Baker, PhD[a,f]

KEYWORDS

- Consumer sleep technology • Wearables • Performance • Health • Sensors

KEY POINTS

- Consumer sleep technologies (CSTs) are largely unregulated. Understanding the rationale behind the technology, the challenges, and the limitations of CSTs is critical for an informed and proper adoption of these technologies in research and clinical applications.
- CSTs have a growing number of sensor capabilities, with multisensory devices having the potential of advancing the accuracy in sleep tracking and also enabling assessment of the functioning of other body systems, such as autonomic functioning.
- CSTs have the potential to advance understanding of sleep and its importance in health, disease, safety, and human performance.

INTRODUCTION

Sleep is a fundamental human need supporting the proper functioning of mind and body.[1–7] Being able to measure and accurately quantify sleep is critical to characterize the sleep processes supporting health and those implicated in disease as well as to understand how and to what extent sleep (a modifiable behavior) can be enhanced to promote healthy living, mitigate or slow the occurrence of clinical conditions, and improve cognitive functioning and performance.

The current gold standard for measuring sleep is polysomnography (PSG), a multichannel recording of scalp cortical brain activity, muscle tone, and eye movement activity (see Kryger and colleagues[8]). To clinically evaluate the presence of sleep disorders, PSG also may include other signals, such as the measurement of airflow and respiratory efforts, leg movements, oxygen saturation, snoring, and body position. PSG is used mainly in the laboratory setting and, occasionally, in nonlaboratory environments (ambulatory PSG). PSG allows an in-depth characterization of sleep physiology, from the sleep macrostructure (the dynamics of wake and sleep stage distribution across the night via manual standard classification of sleep/wake and sleep stages across the night) to a finer analysis of specific features of

Funding: This study was supported by the National Institutes of Health (NIH) grants R01 HL139652 (M. de Zambotti), U01DA041022 (F.C. Baker), and AA021696 (F.C. Baker & I.M. Colrain). N. Cellini was supported by the University of Padova under the STARS Grants program. The content is solely the responsibility of the authors and does not necessarily represent the official views of the National Institutes of Health.

a Center for Health Sciences, SRI International, 333 Ravenswood Avenue, Menlo Park, CA 94025, USA; b Department of General Psychology, University of Padua, Via Venezia, 8 - 35131 Padua, Italy; c Department of Biomedical Sciences, University of Padua, Via Ugo Bassi 58/B - 35121 Padua, Italy; d Padova Neuroscience Center, University of Padua, Via Giuseppe Orus, 2, 35131 Padua, Italy; e Human Inspired Technology Center, University of Padua, Via Luzzatti, 4 - 35121 Padua, Italy; f Brain Function Research Group, School of Physiology, University of the Witwatersrand, 1 Jan Smuts Avenue, Braamfontein 2000, Johannesburg, South Africa
* Corresponding author.
E-mail addresses: massimiliano.dezambotti@sri.com; maxdeze@gmail.com

Sleep Med Clin 15 (2020) 1–30
https://doi.org/10.1016/j.jsmc.2019.11.003
1556-407X/20/© 2019 Elsevier Inc. All rights reserved.

sleep, via the quantitative analysis of cortical electro-encephalographic (EEG) signals.[8] Despite the vision of sleep as a central nervous system (CNS) phenomenon (a state of brain activation), it is important to understand that overall physiology goes through sleep.[9] Although not used for classic standard sleep scoring, additional biosignals can be collected simultaneously as part of PSG and can provide information about the state of bodily systems at night as well as serving as peripheral correlates of cortical events (eg, arousals) and the clinical manifestation of sleep disorders (eg, transient respiratory events). Among the additional signals, the most commonly recorded is the electrocardiogram (ECG), from which beat-to-beat heart rate (HR) can be extracted and its variability quantified as an indication of cardiac autonomic nervous system (ANS) functioning (see de Zambotti and colleagues[9]). Beat-to-beat blood pressure, respiratory rate, skin conductance, and body temperature also can be collected. Thus, PSG can truly offer a complete, detailed picture of the physiologic state of sleep.

Outside the laboratory, actigraphy is considered as the accepted alternative to PSG.[10] Actigraphy can measure objective day-to-day variation in an individual's sleep/wake activity, which, for example, allows understanding of whether an individual sleeps more during the weekend compared with weekdays, potential seasonal variations in sleep, regularities/abnormalities in bed times and rising times, how sleep varies across different geolocations, and so forth. Actigraphy provides an indirect measure of sleep, a crude estimation of an individual sleep/wake patterns by using a motion sensor, usually embedded in a wristwatch, to estimate patterns of motion and classify periods as wake or sleep. Compared with PSG, actigraphy is limited in detecting wake, particularly when sleep is highly disrupted or in the presence of sleep disturbances and in situations in which people are lying in bed but not moving. In those cases, actigraphy misclassifies wake as sleep (for limitations and use of actigraphy, see Sadeh[10]).

Both PSG and actigraphy are research/clinical tools, and their applicability on a large scale is limited, having a relatively high cost, using specialized equipment including dedicated software platforms for data analysis, and requiring specific expertise and trained personnel to operate them.

With the recent boom in new consumer sleep technologies (CSTs), possibly due to advancements in sensor capabilities, communication protocols (eg, Bluetooth), data analysis techniques, data storage (eg, cloud environment), and meeting the consumer market demand for devices of low cost, low power consumption, and small size, it is now becoming possible to track users' behaviors, physiology, and sleep 24/7 with minimal obtrusiveness.

CSTs have several limitations, however. Data usually are extracted via proprietary algorithms that have not been independently validated. Limited validation exists for the summary post-processed data, and no current validation exists on the direct sensor outputs of CSTs, with companies currently not releasing raw data. Users can access their summary data via dedicated mobile app or Internet-based platforms. Some third-party services (eg, Fitabase) aiming at a more clinical/research use of CSTs, do exist and simplify study implementation, data collection, and monitoring: post-processed data can be obtained with a greater time resolution (eg, 30-s epochs), and there is some control on the CSTs algorithm used (algorithm version), although raw data are still not provided. Some CSTs companies also provide an open application programming interface, which allows a more advanced use of wearable operating systems despite not directly accessing the sensors' readings.[11]

CSTs usually are wristwatches or other wearable types of devices (clips, rings, and so forth) with embedded accelerometer and/or additional sensors (eg, photoplethysmography (PPG), temperature, and skin conductance sensors [discussed later]). Noncontact CSTs also exist (termed, *nearables*) and there is a new emerging line of wearables based on the recordings of EEG signals using dry electrodes. Although development of these devices is on the rise, they still do not reach high numbers of users and, to date, are still far from large-scale implementation and usefulness in the field of sleep and circadian science.[11]

CSTs now are widely used by the general population and increasingly used in clinical and research studies (mainly viewed as an alternative to standard actigraphy), linking CST-measured sleep (eg, sleep duration) and sleep-related outcomes (eg, night-time resting HR) with several biopsychosocial factors, performance, and behaviors. Despite recognizing the potential of CSTs, it is important to realize that CSTs pose critical challenges for their implementation in science given the unregulated and uncontrolled nature of an industry product.

There are a growing number of initiatives aimed at providing standards and regulations in using CSTs. In a recent review, de Zambotti and colleagues highlighted the performance, use, and challenges of these devices in the field of sleep and circadian science, by introducing guidelines on how to evaluate and use CSTs.[11] The American Academy of Sleep Medicine (AASM) recently published a position statement warning about the challenges in using CSTs and setting a high bar for their adoption in sleep medicine as a diagnostic tool.[12] A summary of the 2018 International Biomarkers Workshop on Wearables in Sleep and

Circadian Science promoted by the Sleep Research Society also has been released.[13] The expert panel's recommendations include best practices and guidelines for evaluating and using CSTs. The Consumer Technology Association recently released some standards for CSTs, which include definitions of terminology and methods for calculating basic sleep metrics and features used in sleep tracking.[14–16] Importantly, the Food and Drug Administration (FDA) launched a precertification program (Software Precertification Pilot Program, https://www.fda.gov/medical-devices/digital-health/digital-health-software-precertification-pre-cert-program), a new regulatory model to face the rapid expansion of digital health technology on the market that can potentially "replace the need for a premarket submission in some cases and allow for decreased submission content and/or faster review of marketing applications for software products in other cases." Some of the major players in the CSTs (eg, Fitbit and Apple) currently are involved in the FDA precertification program. This new model focuses more on the developer rather than the product per se and allows the public to provide inputs on the program through an open public docket (https://www.regulations.gov/comment?D=FDA-2017-N-4301-0001).

From a scientific point of view, it is fundamental to understand whether and under which circumstances outcomes from CSTs can be trusted and, therefore, how to interpret outcomes from studies already adopting these consumer devices. This review highlights the rationale and the capability behind wearable sleep trackers and describes what wearable sensors can truly record and the meaning of the derived physiologic measures. Finally, a general overview of the current use and potential use of CSTs to investigate relationships between sleep, health, and performance is provided, considering their limitations due to potential errors in sleep quantification.

CONSUMER SLEEP TECHNOLOGIES: SENSORS CAPABILITY AND PHYSIOLOGIC MEANING OF BIOSIGNALS

Rudimental versions of CST sensors have been used since the second half of the past century to monitor the functioning of different physiologic systems (see Holter[17]) and behaviors, such as physical activity, outside the laboratory/clinical setting.

In the context of sleep monitoring, a first motion-based generation of sleep trackers (ie, using accelerometry to estimate patterns of motion and sleep/wake) and a second multisensory generation (ie, using a combination of accelerometry and other features extracted by different biosignals to improve

the detection of sleep/wake patterns and sleep stages) can be distinguished. The newer generation of multisensory CSTs aims to collect information about sleep macrostructure, specifically about wake, light (commonly referred as PSG N1 + N2), deep (commonly referred as PSG N3), and rapid eye movement (REM) sleep (see de Zambotti and colleagues[11]), providing users with a day-by-day feedback on their sleep, sleep-related physiology, and fitness. In most cases, sleep trackers can measure motion and the night-time plethysmography signal, with some of them also collecting information about skin/body temperature and electrodermal activity (skin conductance). This article provides a summary of the main types of physiologic signals the CSTs are capable of collecting for sleep measurement, along with an overview of the physiologic meaning of these signals, processing pipelines, and related challenges (**Table 1**, **Fig. 1**). For a more exhaustive overview on signals used in sleep analysis, see the article by Roebuck and colleagues.[18]

The multisensory capability of the new generation of CSTs has the potential to (1) theoretically, advance the accuracy in sleep tracking by enhancing the capability of algorithms for sleep/wake patterns and sleep stage detection—this is possible thanks to a combination of motion with a broad range of features obtained from different biosignals showing sleep stage–dependent changes (the most common features used by CSTs for sleep tracking are based on the analysis of HR and its variability)—and (2) enable assessment of the functioning of other body systems (eg, cardiac ANS function) during sleep, making a more naturalistic investigation of processes like restoration and recovery possible, as well as the detection of abnormalities in cardiac rhythms, potentially expanding their use as diagnostic tools. See Matar and colleagues[19] for a schematic overview of the physiologic changes (HR and its variability, respiratory pattern, and motion) occurring when transitioning between PSG-defined sleep stages. See also articles by de Zambotti and colleagues,[9,11] Willemen and colleagues,[20] and Faust and colleagues[21] for further details about ANS dynamics during sleep and development and performance of automatic algorithms for measuring sleep/wake and sleep stages based on CNS and ANS information. For instance, Willemen and colleagues[20] used features of cardiorespiratory and movement signals to discriminate sleep stages, reaching an accuracy ranging from 69% (wake-REM-N1N2-N3; Cohen kappa = .56) to 92% (sleep/wake; Cohen kappa = .69). Similarly, Herlan and colleagues[22] constructed an algorithm to discriminate wake and sleep based on skin conductance level (SCL) and skin conductance responses (SCRs), reaching an

Table 1
Consumer sleep technologies: sensors, techniques, and biosignals used in for sleep measurement and quantification

	Signals and Physiologic Meaning	Biosensors and Measurement	Signal Processing and Real-time Processing	Confounders and Challenges	Relevant Post-processed Metrics
Motion/activity	Physical activity can be defined as any type of bodily movement produced by the skeletal muscles and resulting in energy expenditure.[26] Physical activity and body movements are recorded most commonly in terms of acceleration (ie, change in speed over time), expressed in gravitational acceleration units (1g = 9.81 m/s²), using a sampling frequency in the human motion range, for example, between 1 Hz and 25 Hz.[27] Physical activity intensity (eg, low, moderate, and vigorous) can be expressed in activity counts per minute using predefined cutoff points.[28]	Acceleration due to body movements, specifically during sleep, is mainly measured using wrist-mounted, waist-mounted, or hip-mounted accelerometers. In sleep research, nondominant wrist sites have shown better accuracy than other locations.[29] The small size and light weight of wrist-worn accelerometers make them ideal tools for long-term 24 h/d monitoring.[30] Activity monitors may include 1 (monoaxial) to 3 (triaxial) accelerometers, typically consisting of a piezoelectric element whose deformations are converted into proportional voltage changes.[27]	Several validated proprietary (eg, Philips Respironics [Bend, Oregon]) and publicly available algorithms (see Van Hees and colleagues[31] and Sadeh and colleagues[32]) have been proposed to obtain a binary classification (ie, 1 = sleep and 0 = wake) of activity epochs, congruent with PSG. Signal processing includes band-pass filtering (removal of irrelevant types of movement [eg, higher than 25 Hz]), rectification (eg, signal conversion into absolute values), and integration (conversion into digital raw counts at a prefixed frequency). The resulting signal is averaged or summed over time epochs (usually 1 min) to be expressed in terms of "activity counts."[27] Each epoch's value is compared with a predefined threshold	The main limitation in sleep monitoring through actigraphy is due to the definition of sleep as a lack of movement. This implies that motionless wake intervals are classified incorrectly as sleep (low specificity), leading to overestimated TST and SE, and to underestimated SOL and WASO, especially in individuals with sleep disturbances.[10] Further limitations concern the inability to discriminate sleep stages,[34] several sources of artifacts (eg, active bed partner, waterbed, movement disorders), and the need of sleep logs to determine the time window within which motionless intervals are interpreted as sleep.[30,35]	Epochs scored as sleep and wake can be used to compute widely assessed sleep parameters, such as TST, SE, SOL, and WASO, as well as number of awakenings, matching the standard guidelines of the AASM for calculating the standard PSG parameters in both nonclinical and clinical settings.[36] Actigraphy also can be used to objectively estimate TIB. Although self-report information is still the most used method to determine bedtime and wake-up time, some algorithms (see van Hees and colleagues[37]) have recently been proposed to detect these time intervals. The same information may be used to understand potential circadian alterations in sleep timing. On a different time scale, the night-to-night

variability in sleep measures (eg, standard deviation) could be an important metric to consider, because it reflects the regularity of sleep/wake patterns, and it is particularly useful in the context of insomnia disorders.[38] A composite measure has been proposed based on a combination of SOL, TST, WASO, and number of awakenings in order to provide an objective index of sleep disturbance and to discriminate good sleepers and insomniacs (the discriminant score).[39]

(eg, 20 counts) on which the epoch is scored as wake, and under which it is scored as sleep. In most commercial actigraphs, the signal processing is automatically performed by the sensor's firmware and only a summary of activity/sleep metrics is presented to the user (see Albinali and colleagues[33]).

Cardiac function (ECG)	The ECG is the biosignal measured by the surface recording of the cardiac electrical activity.[40] In the ECG, heart cycles are represented by patterns of electric potentials ranging from tenths of microvolts to more than 1 mV. Each potential represents a specific event occurring in the heart: the atrial depolarization (P wave), the ventricular depolarization (QRS	A 12-lead ECG is the standard configuration used in cardiology,[41] but more basic ECG configurations require 2 electrodes plus a ground electrode (usually Ag/AgCl) placed on proximal (chest) or distal sites (arms and legs). Portable ECGs have been used since the 1960s.[17] Modern wireless ECG sensors simply require 2 dry electrodes placed on the chest (see Parak	The heart periods are estimated by measuring the time intervals (milliseconds) between consecutive R peaks (RR intervals or IBIs). Several algorithms (see Benitez and colleagues[46]) have been proposed for an accurate detection of the R-wave peaks in order to precisely measure IBIs. The IBI time series is the raw signal from which HR and HRV metrics are	Artifacts in the ECG signal originate mainly from movements, technical failures or ectopic beats (eg, arrhythmia), resulting in spurious quantifications of IBIs (eg, missing or double beats) and, thus, into biased estimations of HR and HRV metrics.[40] Various artifact detection algorithms, usually based on adaptive and moving thresholds, have been proposed (see	ECG is the gold standard method for measuring HR and HRV, with the latter representing variations in heart periods over time.[45] HR and HRV originate from autonomic innervations of the sinus-atrial node, with vagally mediated cholinergic synapses exerting a tonic inhibitory effect on HR.[40] HRV metrics are derived from the IBI time series and frequently expressed

(continued on next page)

Table 1
(continued)

Signals and Physiologic Meaning	Biosensors and Measurement	Signal Processing and Real-time Processing	Confounders and Challenges	Relevant Post-processed Metrics
complex), and its repolarization (T wave).[40]	and colleagues[42]), making them suitable to be implemented into smart wearable clothes (see Grossman[43]). Similarly, electrodes are embedded into chest belts for HR monitors.[44] Although a sampling rate of $\geq$250 Hz is recommended to detect R waves, a lover sampling rate ($\geq$100 Hz) may still be used with appropriate interpolation techniques.[45]	computed. Instantaneous HR is simply computed by converting the IBIs' length into frequency expressed in beats per minute (instantaneous HR = 1/IBI × 60,000). In cases of HR monitors, such algorithms may be included in the device firmware and the user can be provided with a real-time update—in most cases with a slight delay—of his/her HR (see Ruha and colleagues[47]).	Berntson and colleagues[48]) and implemented into signal processing software (see Kaurmann and colleagues[49]). Thus, the main challenge for HR monitors and ECG-based wearable sensors is to detect artifacts with an acceptable accuracy. A combination of automatic and manual procedures is recommended.[50] Overall, in the analysis of HRV, any potential factors leading to phasic (eg, a sudden sound) and/or tonic (eg, β-blockers) cardiac oscillations within the frequency range of interest (0–0.4 Hz), potentially can invalidate the physiologic meaning of the HRV metrics of interest.	through variability statistics, such as the root mean square of successive differences in IBIs, expressed in milliseconds. Alternative analyses may be performed on the power spectrum density of the IBIs time series, using time-to-frequency transformations (eg, fast Fourier transform) to estimate the power associated with different frequency bands. In particular, HRV in the high frequency range (0.15–0.4 Hz) is considered as an index of vagal cardiac control.[45] Sleep is characterized by marked decreases in HR and increases in vagally mediated HRV, with several studies showing different HRV patterns depending on sleep stages, arousals, awakenings and body movements, and HRV

					synchrony with EEG activity (see de Zambotti and colleagues[9]). Consequently, the unobtrusive monitoring of HRV using CSTs may represent an unique opportunity to investigate sleep patterns and sleep quality (see Fonseca and colleagues[51]), with HRV-type features among the key features used by current CSTs to classify wake, sleep, and sleep stages.
Cardiac function (plethysmogram)	Graphical representations of blood volume variations are called plethysmograms, and when the signal is derived using a photoelectric detector it is called PPG.[40] Thus, PPG is the biosignal reflecting oscillations in the amount of light absorbed by the blood vessels. These oscillations are proportional to changes in the blood volume pulse, with greater blood volume resulting in higher light absorption and lower light reflection. The	A standard PPG sensor uses a light source to illuminate the tissue and a photodetector to record variations in the reflected light intensity. The light source typically uses red or green light-emitting diodes, because shorter wavelengths are more strongly absorbed by skin melanin.[54] The finger is the most commonly used site of PPG measurement, as in the case of pulse oximetry in clinical settings[52] (PPG-derived pulse oximetry uses red and infrared light	Regular features in the PPG waveform (usually the systolic peak or its onset) are used to measure pulse rate intervals (ie, time distances between consecutive pulse peaks) for computing HR and HRV measures.[25] When focusing on the pulsatile (AC) component, preprocessing procedures include filtering, smoothing, and detrending of blood volume pulse raw data.[57] Real-time signal processing is often included in most	The same sources of artifacts and recommendations made for ECG-derived HR and HRV measures also applies to PPG signals, with motion artifacts recognized as the most critical, especially in peripheral measurement sites.[59] Furthermore, the agreement between ECG-derived and PPG-derived HRV metrics depends on physiologic processes, such as the pulse transit time (ie, the delay between a given R wave and the corresponding pulse	In most PPG applications, the pulsatile AC component is used to measure pulse rate and its variability as surrogates of HR and HRV (for a review, see the article be Schäfer and Vagedes[25]). Thus, PPG data can be used to potentially assess sleep patterns as in the case of ECG (see Beattie and colleagues[61] and Fonseca and colleagues[62]). In addition to pulse intervals, other features of the PPG waveform (eg, the systolic peak amplitude, the ratio

(continued on next page)

Table 1
(continued)

Signals and Physiologic Meaning	Biosensors and Measurement	Signal Processing and Real-time Processing	Confounders and Challenges	Relevant Post-processed Metrics
PPG signal includes a pulsatile (AC) component around 1 Hz, depending on heart periods, and a superimposed lower varying (DC) component attributed to changes in RR, sympathetic activity and thermoregulation.[52] The typical PPG waveform shows a first positive peak corresponding to the systole, followed by a negative peak (dicrotic notch), and a third positive peak corresponding to the diastole[53] (**Fig. 2**).	frequencies to estimate blood oxygen saturation, Spo$_2$, in peripheral blood vessels[55]). PPG, however, can be applied to several sites of the body, such as earlobes, forehead, arms, and wrists, with wristband PPG among the most used by CSTs sensors.[56]	commercial PPG CSTs, which are able to show beat-to-beat instantaneous pulse rate or, more frequently, average pulse rate values computed over time windows of a few seconds (see Spierer and colleagues[58]).	wave), which is affected by both dispositional (eg, blood pressure, arterial stiffness, and age) and situational variables (eg, respiratory effort and mental stress).[25] Finally, environmental factors influencing vasodilation, such as ambient temperature, also may lead to biased measures.[60] This is extremely important when considering that PPG-derived HR and HRV metrics are among the features used by CSTs to classify wake, sleep, and sleep stages.	between the 2 areas separated by the dicrotic notch inflection) may provide useful information to improve sleep stage classification.[63] Currently, time spent in light, deep, and REM sleep have become common metrics calculated from the new generation of multisensory CSTs by mainly combining motion-like and PPG features. Deep sleep information, in particular, potentially is useful to quantify homeostatic pressure and its night-time dissipation. Limited evidence, however, supports the accuracy of CSTs in estimating these measures (see de Zambotti and colleagues[11]). Finally, the DC component may be used to estimate patterns of respiration (leading to paced

changes in blood volume pulse amplitude), vasodilation, and sympathetic-induced vasoconstriction (eg, in association with sleep arousals) to provide a more complete overview of the autonomic activity while sleeping.[52] PPG also might be used to indicate whether an individual is wearing the device or not.

Respiration	The respiratory system is a complex network of structures including muscles (eg, diaphragm) and airways (eg, trachea and larynx) through which the oxygenated air reaches the lungs, where it is exchanged with carbon dioxide (see Cacioppo and colleagues[40]). Although several respiratory parameters (eg, air flow rate, lung volume, gas exchange, breathing temperature) can be measured, noninvasive, measures of RR (expressed in cycles per minute), inhalation and exhalation duration,	RR may be measured using noncontact-based (eg, optical, thermal, or radar sensors) or contact-based techniques (eg, nasal microphones and thermistors).[64] Among the latter, common wearable monitors are PPG sensors and respiratory belts. Respiratory belts measure increases in thoracic/abdominal volume due to inhalations using a variety of techniques, such as strain gauges, mercury-filled tubes, inductive coils, and piezoelectric devices.[40]	The data obtained through respiratory belts require only relatively simple processing procedures, such as band-pass filtering the signal (eg, 6–40 cycles per minute) to remove artifacts due to movements unrelated to respiration.[65] In contrast, the RR estimation from pulse intervals requires more complex procedures.[66] Most algorithms doing these procedures are based on the existing relationship between HR and respiration (ie, RSA). Because RSA diminishes in some	Biased measures derived from thoracic or abdominal belts may rise mainly from ceiling effects and loss of data due to tight and large belt fitting, respectively.[40] To prevent these problems, calibration techniques have been suggested.[65] PPG-derived respiratory measures are affected by the same sources of artifacts (eg, movements), described previously.	Besides RR, several respiratory metrics may be computed in both the time (eg, inspiratory and expiratory duration, inspiration/expiration ratio) and frequency domain (spectral analysis).[40] In sleep monitoring, RR has been used for discriminating sleep stages, with non-REM sleep (in particular, deep sleep) characterized by more stable and regular respiratory amplitude and frequency, and other morphologic and variability features have shown to provide

(continued on next page)

Table 1
(continued)

	Signals and Physiologic Meaning	Biosensors and Measurement	Signal Processing and Real-time Processing	Confounders and Challenges	Relevant Post-processed Metrics
	and respiratory effort are among the most commonly used in psychophysiology and sleep research.		conditions (eg, stress, exercise, and in the elderly), however, other strategies focus on the DC component of the PPG signal.[67]		useful information.[20,51,68] Moreover, when recorded simultaneously with IBIs, RSA estimates may be used as a parasympathetic indicator (see Cacioppo and colleagues[40]). Finally, clinical applications, such as RR and Spo2 monitoring for the assessment of OSA, is of growing use and may have clinical utility.[69]
ST	ST is the temperature (in degrees Celsius [°C] or Fahrenheit [°F]) recorded on the skin surface, reflecting both the CT and the peripheral hemodynamic status.[70] CT is the result of several thermoregulatory processes mediated by central and peripheral thermosensory neurons and thermoeffectors (for a review, see Romanovsky[71]). CT typically ranges between 36.5°C and	Thermometers can be classified according to their degree of invasiveness and contact required. Invasive methods, such as oral and rectal sensors, are used for CT measurement.[70] In contrast, ST can be measured through noninvasive methods, such as surface thermistors (transductors whose resistance is sensitive to temperature changes), and noncontact	Depending on the type of thermometer and its sampling rate, different calibration and preprocessing procedures (eg, low-pass filtering) are necessary to obtain the ST time series (see Shusterman and colleagues[75] and Keränen and colleagues[79]). Mean ST values can be computed over time intervals (eg, 1 min), and several formulas may be applied to estimate	ST is affected by several confounding factors, including hemodynamic dysfunction, medications, and environmental temperature.[73] For instance, mean ST measures have shown to be biased by cool environments and subjects wearing heavy clothes.[81] In the case of sleep, the heat flow to the environment may be limited by the use of bed covers.[72] When the	Sleep is associated with decreased heat production, increased heat loss and peripheral vasodilation, leading to lower average CT and higher peripheral ST compared with daytime.[72] Consequently, several ST measures can be used in sleep research, such as average body ST,[82] blood flow measures expressed by the distal-proximal ST gradient,[83] and ST phasic decreases due to

	38.5°C, and it expresses the momentary balance between heat production and heat loss.[72] Differently, peripheral ST is a low-varying signal showing spontaneous oscillations between 32°C and 35°C within the 0.01–2.00 Hz range, partially due to blood flow, blood pressure, and respiration.[73–75]	sensors, such as infrared thermopile (using thermocouples to measure temperature-related infrared radiations).[76] Miniaturized wireless digital thermometers (eg, iButtons [iButtonLink, LLC, Whitewater, WI, USA]) also are increasingly used, especially in sleep research, with the main advantage of allowing simultaneous recordings of ST over multiple sites.[77] Different sites are affected by different sources of heat, with proximal ST (measured on the trunk and the proximal limb parts) more affected by CT, and distal/peripheral ST (measured on the feet, toes, hands, fingers, and ears) out of phase with CT and more affected by blood flow and environmental temperature.[78]	mean ST by weighting the values recorded over multiple sites (see Choi and colleagues[80]). Finally, spectral analyses also have been proposed to distinguish sources of ST variability (cardiac output, respiration, and so forth), although small ST variations may not be distinguishable from external thermal noise.[74]	sensor is embedded in CSTs, the recorded temperature may be affected by the device itself and the included sources of heat.[79]	sympathetically mediated vasoconstriction.[73] Wrist ST has been suggested as a promising index of circadian rhythms, because it showed relatively marked changes concurrent with bedtime and awakening.[84] Moreover, wrist ST sensors increasingly are included in wearable accelerometers to classify wear and non-wear time intervals, providing information on participants' compliance (see Zhou and colleagues[85]).
EDA	EDA is a general term to describe changes in the electrical properties (ie, resistance, potential difference, and conductivity) of the skin surface, as a	Skin conductance measurements are based most commonly on the exosomatic method, using 2 electrodes (usually Ag/AgCl) between which a	Similarly to the previously described signals, a combination of visual inspection and automatic artifacts correction procedures is recommended for	Artifacts in the EDA signal may originate from mechanical pressures on the electrodes, loss of contact (especially with dry electrodes and during ambulatory	When focusing on sleep monitoring, both thermoregulatory and nonthermoregulatory origins of EDA are of interest. Sleep is characterized by ST (in

(continued on next page)

Table 1
(continued)

Signals and Physiologic Meaning	Biosensors and Measurement	Signal Processing and Real-time Processing	Confounders and Challenges	Relevant Post-processed Metrics
function of the secretory activity of eccrine sweat glands.[40,86] Whereas thermoregulation is the primary function of eccrine gland activity, phasic EDA measures, such as SCRs and NS-SCRs, are widely used as indices of sympathetically mediated arousal.[87] Skin conductance is expressed in microsiemens or micromho. Similarly to ST, it varies in a low-frequency range, typically showing 1 to 3 NS-SCRs whose amplitude frequently ranges from 0.1 μsiemen to 1.0 μsiemen and whose latency frequently falls between 1 s and 3 s.[40,86]	weak constant voltage (or current) is passed, and the conductance is recorded as the reciprocal of the skin resistance.[88] A sampling frequency of at least 20 Hz is recommended.[89] EDA is usually measured on the nondominant hand, over skin sites showing the highest sweat glands density: the thenar eminences of palms and soles, and the volar surfaces of the phalanges.[90] Wrist EDA is considered to be more affected by thermoregulatory rather than psychophysiologic processes.[86] Although the NaCl or KCl isotonic paste is recommended,[88] dry electrodes also are	processing raw EDA signal.[86] Low-pass filters of approximately 5 Hz may be used to exclude high-frequency noise (see Bach[94]). Then, the tonic (SCL) and the phasic component (SCRs or NS-SCRs) of the signal should be analyzed separately, to avoid overestimating SCL due to ongoing or overlapping SCRs.[94] Several analytical strategies have been proposed for SCRs detection, including trough-to-peak, deconvolution and model-based analyses.[94,95] A major challenge is the implementation of similar procedures into real-time processing algorithms to be	monitoring), environmental temperature, humidity and dryness, and SCRs due to the subject's activity (eg, respiratory effort) or environmental factors (eg, external sounds).[86,96] The measurement site is particularly important, becuase different body locations may show very different patterns of responsiveness.[97] Finally, because reliable EDA measurements require the preservation of the skin electrical properties, simple subjects' actions (eg, hand washing) may introduce noise or attenuate the recorded signal.[40]	particular, wrist ST) increases.[72,84] Coherently, increased SCL and relatively frequent SCL rises (called storms) have been observed, especially in the earlier part of the night,[98] with more pronounced increases in wrist than palmar SCL.[99] Because these rises tend to disappear in REM sleep (during which thermoregulatory processes are inhibited), they have been associated with thermal sweating.[96] It is still unclear if EDA measures may be used for sleep stage classification/differentiation.[22] Other potential uses of EDA should be explored. Variations in

	suitable to record EDA in most cases, and they are increasingly included into CSTs wearable recording systems, including wristbands,[91] gloves,[92] and socks.[93]	implemented in wearable sensors.	sympathetically mediated finger and palmar EDA may be used as indices of presleep and nocturnal arousals, possibly involved in sleep disturbances.[100] Phasic fluctuations in wrist EDA have been used in combination with motion features for seizure detection.[101] Wearable SCL signals also could be useful for hot flash detection. A hot flash is a heat dissipation response characterized by cutaneous vasodilation and sweating, a hallmark of the menopausal transition, objectively recorded by changes in sternum SCL (SCL rise >2 μsiemen within 30 s). Hot flashes can be particularly disrupting at night, being associated with awakening and CV surges.[102,103]
Environmental light	Light is particularly critical for all circadian processes, particularly for sleep. Light exposure is the most — Light exposure may be measured in terms of illuminance (1 lux = 1 lumen/m²), color temperature (in kelvins)	Sensor light usually can process wavelengths in the range of 400–1100 nm, with different intensity, depending on	Although light detection may be relatively easy to perform in some applications involved in sleep monitoring, when — Light recorded during sleep monitoring is useful to improve sleep detection. Actigraphy-based sleep scoring *(continued on next page)*

Table 1
(continued)

Signals and Physiologic Meaning	Biosensors and Measurement	Signal Processing and Real-time Processing	Confounders and Challenges	Relevant Post-processed Metrics
important environmental cue (zeitgeber) that regulates circadian rhythms in mammals.[104,105] Light quantification also can be useful to evaluate the relation between light exposure and sleep. For instance, diurnal bright light treatments have shown positive effects on sleep quality,[106] whereas environmental light during sleep time and lack of synchronization between light exposure and the endogenous clock have been associated with poorer sleep quality.[107,108]	and spectral power distribution. In sleep research, light exposure is mostly measured using standard equipment for illuminance (eg, luxmeters, photodiodes, and other photo detectors) and light color detection (eg, photo radiometers). Because the circadian and the visual system are affected by different lighting features,[109] however, the use of calibrated devices for measuring person-specific light exposure has been recommended in this field of research.[107] For instance, a head-worn device (the Daysimeter; see Miller and colleagues[110]) using	the type of sensor (see Kamisalic and colleagues[112]). Some sensors are specific for different wavelengths (eg, blue spectrum: 400–500 nm, green spectrum: 500–600 nm, red spectrum: 600–700 nm), allowing to analyze differences in the environmental light. Other sensors have been developed to measure ultraviolet lights (290–400 nm). Several measures can be derived from these sensors, for example, intensity, duration, and timing of light exposure. In most applications, where only light intensity is measured, environmental light is recorded directly by the sensor and converted to	the light detector is contained into a wearable sensor the measurement may be affected by several factors. For instance, a major problem of wrist-worn light detectors is the occlusion by long sleeves and bed linens. Consequently, the light sensors should be directed outward and set for maximal sensitivity to light (see Borazio and colleagues[113]).	relies on the determination of sleep time periods, usually defined as the time between lights-off and lights-on. Self-report sleep diaries often are used to determinate these times, but light (as well as potentially the use of event markers and to some extent ST) can be used as adjunctive information for determining individual bedtime and wake-up times. Several light features may be taken into account when investigating the role of light on sleep and circadian functioning. These include the light quantity (ie, illuminance), spectrum, spatial distribution,

photosensors, accelerometers, and temperature sensors have been developed to study circadian activity and light exposure.[110] Nevertheless, these types of sensors may not be ideally comfortable for long-term continuous sleep monitoring. As an alternative, wearable devices measuring ambient light through small embedded sensors (eg, photodiodes[111]) might be preferred.

current or voltage. Light intensity is averaged over epochs of time based on the device sampling frequency. Alternatively, the information can be encoded using a binary classification (ie, light on/light off) similarly to actigraphic classification.

timing, and duration.[109] Specific metrics to investigate circadian processes also have been proposed, such as the phasors, representing the magnitude and phase relationship between behavioral (ie, activity-rest) and light data (ie, light-dark) measured by the same sensor.[110,114]

Abbreviations: CT, core body temperature; EDA, electrodermal activity; IBI, interbeat interval; NS, nonspecific; RR, respiratory rate; RSA, respiratory sinus arrhythmia; SCL, skin conductance level; SOL, sleep-onset latency; ST, skin temperature; TIB, time spent in bed; WASO, wake after sleep onset.

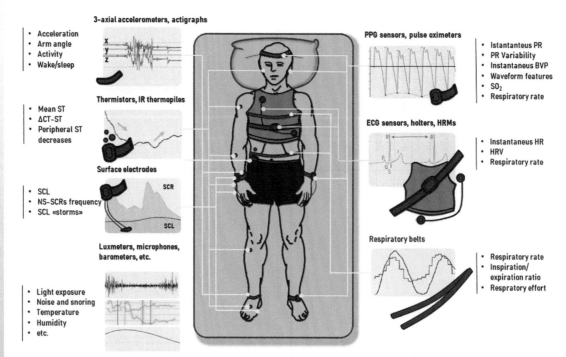

Fig. 1. Critical signals provided by Consumer Sleep Technologies (CSTs) wearable sensors for measuring sleep. BVP, blood volume pulse; CT, core temperature; ECG, electrocardiogram; HR, heart rate; HRM, heart rate monitor; HRV, heart rate variability; IR, infra-red; NS-SCRs, non-specific skin conductance responses; PPG, photoplethysmogram; PR, pulse rate; SCL, skin conductance level; SO2, blood oxygen saturation; ST, skin temperature.

overall accuracy of 86% (97% sensitivity and 75% specificity).

Although there is a strong theoretic basis for applying a multidimensional approach to sleep staging, it is challenging for CSTs to implement this approach for several reasons. CSTs target gold-standard PSG-level accuracy, whereas (1) PSG is based on experts' manual-visual scoring of sleep records and (2) PSG does not provide an absolute reference point.[11] For example, high and variable levels of agreement between experts in scoring sleep records (usually highest for REM sleep and wake, followed by N3 and N2 sleep, with the poorest agreement for N1 sleep) exist and may pose severe challenges for algorithm development.[23] Furthermore, although methodological guidelines for validating CSTs have begun to appear (see de Zambotti and colleagues[11] and Depner and colleagues[13]), specific academic standards for validation metrics (eg, threshold for accuracy for sleep and wake classification) currently do not exist.

The use of ANS signals to estimate CNS (EEG)-based sleep staging is still in its infancy, even within the academic field. ANS-based sleep staging relies on the complex and still largely unexplored sleep CNS-ANS dynamics,[9] and the current performance of academic-based automatic algorithms using 1 or more laboratory-grade peripheral signals (respiration, motion, and ECG) as well as when based on

automatic analysis of EEG signals do not fully match PSG-level manual sleep staging.[20,21,24] The use of commercial sensors from CSTs adds further complexity. For example, common ANS metrics used by CSTs for sleep staging, that is, HR variability (HRV) features, may differ according to whether they are obtained by analyzing the electrical activity of the heart (ECG) or by analyzing blood flow (using a PPG-type sensor).[25] Also, obtaining a high signal-to-noise ratio when using commercial unobtrusive sensors in noncontrolled laboratory conditions is challenged by several potential sources of artifacts due to environmental features (eg, ambient temperature) and other factors (eg, sensor shift) that often cannot be monitored (see **Table 1**).

To date it is still unclear what advancements can be made using peripheral information to classify EEG-based sleep/wake and sleep staging. Improvements in hardware solutions, sensors integration, and signal processing techniques and more collaboration between academia and industry are among the crucial requirements for further advancing the field.

The types of information that CSTs can collect are continuously increasing. For instance, impressive technological advancements have been made in the field of electrochemical sensors able to detect metabolites, electrolytes, and hormones (eg, catecholamines, antioxidants, and cortisol) from sweat, tears, saliva, and skin interstitial fluid.[115] Moreover, other environmental features indexing or influencing sleep patterns and their physiology, such as ambient temperature, humidity, and noise, also are monitored by some devices.[116] CSTs, including microphones for ambient noise measurement, also may be used to assess sleep-related behaviors, such as snoring.[18] A useful feature included in some CSTs is the event marker button, which allows a user to highlight the presence of the stimulus of interest directly within the recording (eg, event markers have been used extensively in actigraphy literature to mark lights-off and lights-on times).[117] Finally, promising developments in data processing (including real-time computation) in all these signals are possible due to the increasing implementation of machine learning techniques, such as random decision forests (see Jeng and colleagues[118]).

ACCURACY OF CONSUMER SLEEP TECHNOLOGIES FOR MEASURING SLEEP AND SLEEP-RELATED OUTCOMES: THE IMPORTANCE OF BIASES IN THE CONTEXT OF BIG DATA

There are a growing but limited number of studies testing the accuracy of CSTs against gold-standard PSG, and these studies used different CST devices (different brands and models), in a variety of different samples (healthy and clinical) and under different conditions (see de Zambotti and colleagues[11] for a detailed review of performance and limitations of sleep-tracking CSTs). These validation studies are performed on post-processed CSTs outcomes; the accuracy of CSTs direct sensor readings is still largely unknown. Overall, CSTs compared with PSG perform better in detecting sleep (higher sensitivity) than wake (relatively lower specificity), with a general tendency to overestimate PSG total sleep time (TST) and underestimate PSG wake time at night. This limitation is in line with the performance of standard actigraphy. The performance of CSTs was not dissimilar from the performance of research/clinical-grade actigraphy in studies in which individuals simultaneously wore CSTs and standard actigraphy and their performance was tested against PSG (see de Zambotti and colleagues[11]). This pattern may change with the new generation of multisensory CSTs, in which the use of sleep-tracking algorithms based on multifeatures is in the early stages and may still have room for improvement.

Evidence indicates that CST devices used with different settings (eg, sensitive mode) than normal had the poorest performance. Moreover, few CST devices have been tested against PSG for accuracy in estimating sleep stages (light, deep, and REM sleep), with the poorest performance for deep sleep

(PSG N3) classification. Distinguishing N3 sleep from N2 sleep even from PSG using AASM rules is challenging: N3 is discriminated from N2 by the visual recognition of a greater presence of slow wave sleep (>20% of the epoch). Possibly, with future advances in knowledge of precise rhythmic changes in peripheral signals, such as HRV linked with sleep stages and/or specific sleep events like slow waves,[9] there may be improvements in CSTs' detection of sleep stages.

Less evidence is currently available for the performance of CSTs in measuring sleep-related physiology. By evaluating a CST wristband, de Zambotti and colleagues previously found that the device underestimated overnight ECG-derived HR by 0.88 beats per minute (bpm), an error that was very small and constant across hours of the night.[119] When testing a similar CST device model in adults,[120] no differences were found between CST-derived HR and ECG-derived HR (0.09 bpm mean difference), although greater levels of error were found in those participants in the lower (<50 bpm) or higher (>80 bpm) ranges of HR.

The access to physiologic metrics on a high temporal resolution (eg, beat-to-beat HR) from CSTs is limited or not available. Thus, the performance of CSTs in measuring sleep-related physiology like sleep HRV is unknown. There are also other potential limitations in CSTs performance, including poor detection of daytime naps, unclear reliability over time, and potential for device failures, as reviewed elsewhere by de Zambotti and colleagues.[11]

Most validation studies are done in the laboratory (using single-night PSG device comparison in convenient samples), which is not the expected setting for using CSTs. Given the impracticality of running at-home PSG validation studies, new paradigms for at-home validation need to be explored. Comparisons between CSTs with standard actigraphy or sleep diaries may provide some insight in the CSTs performance but are questionable as a means of determining CSTs' core validity. Currently, sleep outcomes measured via PSG according to the AASM guidelines[121] should be considered as the only ground truth. A multidisciplinary effort is needed to face this critical barrier.

There is a rapid adoption of CSTs without proper consideration of the implications. Several factors can affect device accuracy, which is particularly critical when using multisensory CSTs. Although alterations to the pattern of motion are responsible for PSG device discrepancies in motion-only–based devices, alterations to 1 or multiple features (eg, motion and autonomic features) used to score wake, sleep, and sleep stages potentially can affect performance in multisensory devices and can have a profound effect on data outcomes. **Table 2** shows

Table 2
Example of factors affecting the biases (level of inaccuracy) of consumer sleep technologies outcomes compared with gold-standard polysomnography

Factors Affecting the Biases	Main Findings for Factors Affecting Consumer Sleep Technologies–Polysomnography Biases (Consumer Sleep Technologies' Level of Inaccuracy in Estimating Sleep)
True (PSG-defined) sleep	Worse true sleep leads to worse CST performance. Evidence suggests a greater bias and/or shifting (from overestimation to underestimation or vice versa) in PSG-CST devices biases and/or greater dispersion of the biases for WASO estimation as a function of increases in PSG WASO. This effect was evident in midlife women with and without a *DSM* (Fourth Edition) insomnia diagnosis (greater device inaccuracy in those women with greater amount of WASO),[122] healthy adults,[123,124] adult patients with unipolar major depressive disorder,[125] adults with insomnia,[126] patients with suspected central disorders of hypersomnolence,[127,128] and healthy adolescents.[119,129]
	In a study of healthy adolescents, investigators found a shifting (from overestimation to underestimation) in PSG-CST device bias for light sleep (N1 + N2) as a function of PSG light sleep.[129] In testing several CST devices in healthy young adults, Mantua and colleagues[130] showed a shifting from underestimation to overestimation of deep (N3) sleep as a function of the PSG deep sleep. In another study, investigators found a shifting from overestimation to underestimation in PSG-CST device biases for deep and REM sleep, as a function of the PSG values of these parameters, in healthy adults.[123] Overall, the dependency of PSG-CST device biases in sleep stages estimation as a function of the amount of time spent in the respective PSG sleep stage seems to be a common finding from the multisensory CSTs (see also Cook and colleagues[127,128]).
	These findings are extrapolated mainly from the interpretation of the Bland-Altman plots and/or regression analyses of the biases.
Demographics	Age affects CSTs performance. In a study testing CST performance in different age groups, investigators found a greater CST wrist-worn device inaccuracy for TST (overestimation ~70 min), WASO (underestimation ~54 min), and SE (overestimation ~14%) in adolescents (13–18 y) compared with school-age (6–12 y) and preschool (3–5 y) children.[131] Similar results were provided by other investigators.[132] In[133] PSG-CST devices, however, discrepancies were greater in prepubertal children (9–11 y) compared with postpubertal adolescents (17–19 y) for WASO (~24 min vs ~13 min) and SE (~5% vs ~3%). It is unclear whether the different pattern was due to the use of a different CST device or to the sample used (in the study by Pesonen and Kuula,[133] adolescents had a higher variability in their sleep compared with children). Within the adolescence period, another study showed a greater and/or shifting (overestimation to underestimation or vice versa) in PSG-CST device biases for TST, WASO, SE, and SOL as a function of age. Overall, there was a greater device inaccuracy in older compared with younger adolescents, in both male and female participants.[134]
	Age and BMI also have been found to be related to PSG-CST device biases for TST and SE (greater overestimation of these measures with advancing age and in those with lower BMI), in a sample of adults with different sleep disorder diagnoses, including breathing-related sleep disorders, hypersomnia, and parasomnia.[135]
Device position	In evaluating the performance of a CST wearable ring in adolescents, the device position affected the performance of the device. PSG device discrepancies for light and REM sleep were significant when individuals were wearing the device on the ring finger compared with the index and the other fingers.[129] It is unclear to what extent factors like sweating, tightness/looseness, and position of the device affect the device accuracy.

(continued on next page)

Table 2 (continued)	
Factors Affecting the Biases	**Main Findings for Factors Affecting Consumer Sleep Technologies–Polysomnography Biases (Consumer Sleep Technologies' Level of Inaccuracy in Estimating Sleep)**
Clinical status	Greater PSG-CST device discrepancies in those individuals with greater severity or presence of sleep disorders. Meltzer and colleagues[136] divided a sample of children and adolescents (3–18 y) based on their sleep AHI to form 3 groups: no OSA (no OSA; AHI <1.5), mild OSA (1.5 ≤AHI ≤5) and moderate/severe OSA (AHI >5). There was a progressive decrease in performance of the CST device as a function of the SDB status, with those categorized as moderate/severe OSA having the poorest performance for TST (overestimation ~76 min), WASO (underestimation ~66 min), and SE (overestimation ~16%) estimation compared with PSG. Although no differences were found according to clinical status for these variables, Toon and colleagues[132] found PSG-CST device differences in SOL estimation (significant underestimation of ~10 min) in children with primary snoring compared with those with mild and moderate/severe OSA. Kang and colleagues[137] found a greater CST device overestimation of PSG TST (~33 min vs ~7 min) and SE (~8% vs ~2%) in adults meeting *DSM* (Fifth Edition) criteria for insomnia disorder compared with good sleepers, with only 39.4% of insomnias vs 82.4% of good sleepers having PSG device biases ≤30 min for TST and ≤5% for SE. Despite the absence of a control group, a pilot study evaluating the performance of CSTs in 7 presymptomatic and early symptomatic Huntington gene carriers found wide PSG-CST device discrepancies for TST (>75 min overestimation) and SE (>15% overestimation).[138]

Abbreviations: AHI, apnea-hypopnea index; *DSM, diagnostic and statistical manual of mental disorders*; SOL, sleep-onset latency; WASO, wake after sleep onset.

some of the potential factors affecting CSTs' accuracy. Factors highlighted in **Table 2** may not be directly responsible for the inaccuracy of CSTs but may reflect other hidden factors (eg, greater device inaccuracy as a function of developmental age may reflect a change in the pattern of motion with age or an age-dependent change in the relation between electrocortical activity and autonomic functioning during the night). It also is important to consider that factors implicated in PSG device inaccuracy may vary in different CST devices models and samples (eg, children vs adults).

Fig. 2 highlights the potential issue of nonconstant biases (different level of error) over time. It is critical to raise awareness that individuals' day-to-day variations in true sleep may be misrepresented by CSTs. It cannot be assumed that the performance of CSTs is always valid and that the same level of accuracy is achieved every day, because conditions vary (eg, sleeping with a bed partner and having a

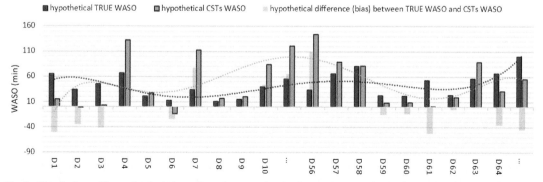

Fig. 2. Simulation of hypothetical sleep data for an individual over time. In the graph, the TRUE day-to-day variation in WASO, a main parameter of interest in sleep research, is provided in red. In gray, the hypothetical WASO obtained from CSTs is displayed by accounting for the randomly generated biases (distance between TRUE WASO and CST-derived WASO), in blue. The level of concordance between TRUE WASO and CSTs WASO changes over time.

variable amount of wake time) and between different people. In the figure, the hypothetical TRUE pattern of sleep in red and the hypothetical wearable pattern in gray have different levels of concordance at different times. The source of inaccuracy could be due to myriad different factors, as described previously, and also could include changes in behavior or condition (eg, caffeine or alcohol consumption, physical exercise, fever, and menstrual cycle phase). These factors may alter not only individual physiology but also the output measures of sleep and other variables CSTs use to score sleep, potentially having an impact on the bias of the device.

In summary, although CSTs hold a lot of promise, there is still a need to further understand their limitations, particularly given the growing use of CSTs in the field, with limited experimental control and generating overwhelming big data sets. These data give incredible power for analyses but high complexity in study outcomes interpretation not only for healthy sleepers but also when using CSTs to track or evaluate a clinical disorder or influence treatment decisions. Understanding the level of accuracy (and of the bias) of a specific CST is particularly critical when considering its potential use in precision medicine and integration in the health care Internet of Things.

POTENTIAL USE OF CONSUMER SLEEP TECHNOLOGIES IN THE CONTEXT OF DISEASE RECOGNITION AND INTERVENTION AND IN GATHERING INSIGHT INTO THE RELATIONSHIPS BETWEEN SLEEP, HEALTH, AND PERFORMANCE

The previous sections discuss the sensors used by CSTs, their limitations, and factors that could affect their performance. Next, the potential of CSTs for use in a wide range of applications is discussed. Although the limitations need to be kept in mind, CSTs hold promise for the continuous passive monitoring of sleep and related physiology, an important step in advancing biomedical research and personalized health.[139] CSTs integrated with ecological momentary assessments (EMAs) (see Bertz and colleagues,[140] Colombo and colleagues,[141] Seppala and colleagues[142] and Shiffman and colleagues[143]), powered by the widespread use of electronic diaries and self-report data collection via mobile technology, allow the study of sleep in relation to a wide range of life factors (eg, physical activity, alcohol consumption, and stress) implicated in sleep health and performance in daily life. The main advantage is the combination of objective and subjective data (multimethod) in real life (ecologically valid), contextualized in time (avoiding recall biases), and over

prolonged periods (longitudinal). Also, toward the push for precision medicine, data-driven approaches to digital phenotyping of specific individuals' health profiles (see Jain and colleagues[144]) could be a reality and lead to enhancement in early detection and management of diseases. Following that, there is a need for different analytical methods and computational skills to deal with the growing amount, variety, and complexity of longitudinal, integrated data sets.

Mobile technology also can be viewed as a tool for implementing intervention, as in the case of cognitive behavioral therapy (CBT) for insomnia (discussed later). In addition, smartphones offer a direct way to communicate with participants (eg, by sending notifications or messages to ensure adherence and protocol compliance) and also could be considered as wearable devices. Smartphones are constantly carried by the users and are capable of providing additional sensory outputs, such as global positioning system geolocation, as well as collecting additional data, such as app usage (eg, social media), call and text message logs (eg, time and duration), and screen usage. Smartphones also have integrated internal sensory capability to quantify relevant metrics among those described in **Table 1** (eg, phone camera can be used to track pulse waveform from an individual's finger and to calculate HRV metrics; snoring episodes can be detected through the microphone).

The next section highlights some of the sleep-relevant areas in which CSTs currently are used. Study outcomes need to be interpreted cautiously when considering that CSTs outcomes may be affected by myriad unpredictable factors having an impact on their accuracy (discussed see **Table 2**, for example). Privacy, security vulnerabilities, and ethical questions also need to be considered.

Health

Sleep is implicated in the regulation of many biological processes, including autonomic, metabolic, immune, and cardiovascular (CV) functioning.[1-6] Wearables, implantable devices, and other type of electronics, including CSTs, are of growing interest for CV monitoring (see Hong and colleagues[145]). The simultaneous continuous collection of sleep (eg, sleep duration[146]), cardiac physiology (eg, resting HR[147]), and integrated data and factors implicated in CV health may lead to better recognition and management of CV disease (CVD) conditions, albeit with the challenge of translating complex big data sets into useful clinical information.

For example, recent results (preprint) from Teo and colleagues[148] showed significant relationships between CST-derived sleep outputs (TST and sleep efficiency [SE]) and several markers of CVD (body mass index [BMI], total cholesterol, resting HR, waist circumference, waist-to-height ratio, and high-density lipoprotein) as well as sample demographics (age, gender, ethnicity, and socioeconomic and lifestyle factors). These relationships were absent when using subjective instead of CST-derived sleep outcomes. Other studies linked CST-derived sleep measures with BMI in adults[149,150] and obesity in adolescence.[151]

The use of wearable technology–based analytical platforms is increasing. For example, Cardiogram (Cardiogram, Inc., San Francisco, CA, USA) applies artificial intelligence (AI) algorithms to data obtained from commercial devices (eg, Apple Watch, Wear OS, Garmin, and Fitbit devices). Initial data collected in collaboration with the University of California, San Francisco (see Health eHeart Study: http://www.health-eheartstudy.org), showed the potential of this approach to screen for several conditions (high cholesterol, diabetes, hypertension, sleep apnea, and atrial fibrillation) associated with elevated CV risk.[152,153] Any effort allowing large-scale affordable early detection of CV risk profiles could be translated in more effective treatments and reductions in the socioeconomic impact of CVDs.

AI (machine learning) applied to CST data (HR cosinor analysis outputs, sleep measures, and activity data) also have been promising in predicting mood state and mood-related episodes (depressive episode, manic episode, hypomanic episode, or no episode), as assessed via self-reported electronic assessments in patients with major depressive and bipolar disorders.[154] These results using continuous passive wearable data collection potentially can expand the capability of previously explored mood prediction models based on mobile built-in sensors. Trained AI algorithms and large data sets available in public repositories may be useful tools to advance the use of AI in precision medicine.

The use of CSTs outcomes has shown to be promising in several other areas of health monitoring and health care, linking CST-derived sleep measures and related physiologic data with a broad range of health outcomes, including self-reported pediatric asthma impact in adolescent patients with asthma,[155] patient-reported outcomes in adult patients with diabetes,[156] and health outcomes in astronauts in an 8-month simulated Mars mission.[157] These results should be viewed cautiously at this early stage of CSTs application, when the need to understand whether CSTs measure true sleep and under which circumstances CSTs measure biases (errors) challenge the validity and interpretation of study outcomes.

Sleep Disorders

In 2003 (and in the 2007 update[36]), the AASM included the use of actigraphy in sleep medicine practice, such as in the assessment of sleep patterns in patients with insomnia, to provide diagnosis of circadian rhythm disorders and to evaluate the outcome of sleep treatments. The same AASM article included several applications in which the use of actigraphy is not recommended, for instance in the diagnosis of sleep-disordered breathing (SDB) or of periodic limb movements. Regarding the use of CSTs, the AASM has clearly stated, "CSTs cannot be utilized for the diagnosis and/or treatment of sleep disorders at this time."[12] Nevertheless, some attempts to test CSTs accuracy in the evaluation of sleep disorders have been made. Although mixed results have been reported for insomnia disorders,[122,158] studies focusing on central disorders of hypersomnolence[127,128] or SDB generally showed that sleep trackers cannot detect, with sufficient accuracy, sleep patterns in these conditions.[132,136,159,160] Moreover, as showed in a recent review,[161] smartphone applications for obstructive sleep apnea (OSA) monitoring cannot fulfill the required standards for diagnosis, even in cases where multiple external sensors (eg, sound, position, and oxygen saturation) are combined.

Although CSTs limitations are clearly emphasized in the published guidelines, the diagnostic accuracy of these devices is continuously improving. For instance, in a recent article, Camci and colleagues[162] developed a prescreening tool to detect respiratory issues during sleep by combining a smartwatch (Gear S3 [Samsung Electronics Co., Ltd., Suwon-si, Korea]) with a microphone app (the Smart Voice Recorder [Smartmob, LLC., Seattle, WA, USA]). Other studies have developed systems to predict apnea events within 1 minute to 3 minutes prior to the event using a wearable multisensory suite, which collects ECG, respiration, heart sounds, and oxygen saturation data.[163] They were able to correctly discriminate 16 out of 17 participants as OSA patients or healthy sleepers. The combination of sleep tracker and smartphone apps also has been tested, with mixed results, as a screening tool for insomnia, to provide Internet-based CBT (iCBT)[158,164–166] or to assess the effect of interventions on sleep patterns.[167,168] Although studies have not yet validated any sleep trackers for circadian rhythm disorder, a recent article described the social jet lag and chronotype in approximately 50,000 individuals wearing a smartwatch.[169]

In summary, although CSTs cannot currently be used for the diagnosis and/or treatment of sleep disorders,[12] further technological improvements may, in the near future, allow their use as a supporting tool for assessing sleep conditions and facilitate online treatments.

Academic Performance

Sleep plays a key role in cognitive functions, and it is consistently shown that its quantity and quality affect academic performance in students of different ages.[170] College students typically have irregular sleep/wake patterns,[171] which is a modifiable factor. In 1 randomized-trial, Chu and colleagues[172] propose a mobile sleep-management learning system based on self-regulated learning strategies to improve sleep quality in undergraduate students. The system is composed of a wearable device (no product name reported) connected to a smartphone app, which provides information, feedback, and tips about a participant's sleep. Participants used the system for 2 weeks and showed self-reported sleep improvement. No academic performance or objective sleep data were reported. Notwithstanding the limitations of this study, a potential application of CSTs is to help students of different ages keep track of their sleep/wake patterns and to provide them feedback or iCBT treatment in order to improve their sleep and, eventually, their academic performance. Another potential application of wearable sensors is to predict academic performance in students. For example, Sano and colleagues[173] collected self-reported and physiologic data (accelerometer, skin conductance, and skin temperature) in 66 college students using a combination of wearable sensors (Q Sensor [Affectiva, Boston, MA, USA]) and smartphone app. Using a machine learning approach, they were able to classify, with 67% to 92% of accuracy (depending on how many features were included), students with high grade point average (GPA) or low GPA. A similar approach, but only based on a smartphone app, was developed by Dartmouth College to successfully predict cumulative GPA in college students.[174]

These studies show the potential of CSTs, alone or in combination with smartphone apps, to modify sleep/wake cycles or to predict academic performance in college students, and, therefore, could be used to plan individualized interventions. These applications, however, also have intrinsic privacy issues that need to be addressed carefully.

Sports Performance

Sleep plays a key role in sports performance. Several observations converge to support the idea that sleep loss and poor sleep quality impair sport performance, whereas good sleep quality seems to improve it.[175] These observations seem particularly important for professional athletes, who often are traveling, playing at night, and participating in competition with tight schedules.[176] Over the past few decades, several interventions have been proposed to deal with the constant circadian shift and reduced time and quality of sleep that athletes experience.[177] In recent years, CSTs have been proposed as a tool to improve sleep in athletes, for example, by providing feedback about sleep.[178] Little investigation has been carried out, however, to assess the reliability and the impact of CSTs on improving sleep and circadian rhythms in athletes (see Sargent and colleagues[179]). Differently, CSTs and other wearable sensors and mobile applications are used to manage athletes' training loads based on the assessment of their physiologic parameters during sleep and immediately after awakening (eg, morning HRV has been found to discriminate overtraining states) (see Plews and colleagues[180]) and mobile applications are increasingly used by professional and amateur athletes to set their own training based on their HRV-derived fitness level and recovery (see Altini and colleagues[181]).

Given the growing number of wearable devices used by the general population as well as elite athletes, there is a need for further studies to investigate the potential usefulness of CSTs as a tool to improve sleep and, consequently, sports performance in athletes.

Work Stress and Performance

Whereas poor sleep quality and sleep disturbances typically are considered consequences of work-related demands and psychosocial factors (for a review, see Linton and colleagues[182]), several multiwave and daily diary studies focused on the reciprocal relationship between sleep and work-related outcomes.[183] For instance, higher-than-usual sleep quality and duration were associated with morning affect (in terms of higher positive activation and serenity and lower negative activation and fatigue) in a sample of 166 employees, controlling for gender, age, position, and trait affect.[184] The recovery model proposed by Demerouti and colleagues[185] identifies sleep quality as the main recovery activity that directly predicts the psychological and energetic states in the morning. In turn, the feeling of being physically and mentally recovered in the morning is positively related to work outcomes, such as daily task performance, personal initiative, and organizational citizenship behavior (see Binnewies[186]).

From a research-oriented perspective, the relationship between sleep and work-related outcomes has been investigated almost exclusively using self-report techniques. Thus, CSTs may offer the opportunity to replicate and integrate these findings using a multimethod approach (eg, CSTs combined with EMAs) more suitable to measure multifaceted phenomena, such as work stress and workplace performance.[187,188] From a more practical point of view, the information collected by these types of sensors embedded in commercially available devices may be used by employers and safety managers to promote employees' health and well-being and optimize the workforce productivity. For instance, some evidence suggests that smartwatch-derived sleep quality may predict so-called fitness to work (eg, psychomotor vigilance and drowsiness).[189]

Recently, a team of researchers at Dartmouth College has developed a classification system that uses information passively recorded by smartphones (eg, location and ambient light), wearable sensors (eg, HRV, physical activity, and sleep) and Bluetooth beacons (eg, time spent at work and number of breaks) to discriminate between lower performers and higher performers.[190] The classifier has been trained and tested against a battery of job performance surveys administered 3 times per week on 554 employees over 2 months to 8.25 months, showing an area under the receiver operating characteristic curve of 0.83. Importantly, several sleep features (eg, light/deep sleep duration and awakenings during sleep) showed different patterns in lower performers and higher performers.

Safety

Another potential application of CSTs is aimed at reducing sleepiness-related errors and injuries. A significant portion of errors made at work is linked (at least subjectively) to sleepiness, sleep problems, and poor sleep hygiene,[191] with shift work and professional driving (see Folkard and colleagues[192]) among the occupations most exposed to safety risks associated with sleep problems.[193] Sleep quality measured using wrist-worn actigraphs was used by Mollicone and colleagues[194] to compute a fatigue scale able to predict drivers' performance and safety (ie, frequency of hard-braking events). A predicting model for driver alertness was proposed by focusing on the circadian variation of CST metrics (eg, HR and HRV).[195,196] The use of wrist-worn wearable data also has been explored to potentially detect instances of distracted driving.[197] Other attempts of using consumer wearable technology to detect driving-related vigilance levels have focused on the use of EEG and/or electrooculography types of signals (see Zheng and colleagues[198]). Overall, this is a promising area of investigation with CSTs, although their usefulness in improving driver safety requires further research.

SUMMARY

CSTs allow longitudinal and real-time monitoring of human physiology and behavior and environmental factors and can be considered an integrated part of the mobile health revolution. The use of CSTs in biomedical research is on the rise and shows great potential in providing new insight into the role of sleep in human functioning in health and disease. The multisensory capability of CSTs and their easy integration with EMAs and other digital technologies could lead to endless possibilities. However, the understanding of functioning, sensor capability, accuracy of CSTs outcomes, is still rudimentary. Also, privacy and ethical implications of CSTs require further attention. These issues need to be addressed in order to properly implement and use CSTs in biomedical research.

ACKNOWLEDGMENTS

The present work was carried out in the scope of the research program "Dipartimenti di Eccellenza" from MIUR (Italian Ministry of Education, University and Research) to the Department of General Psychology.

CONFLICT OF INTEREST

The authors declare no conflict of interest related to the current work. M. de Zambotti and F.C. Baker have received research funding unrelated to this work from Ebb Therapeutics Inc., Fitbit Inc., International Flavors & Fragrances Inc., Verily Life Sciences, LLC, and Noctrix Health, Inc.

REFERENCES

1. Grandner MA. Sleep, health, and society. Sleep Med Clin 2017;12(1):1–22.
2. Besedovsky L, Lange T, Haack M. The sleep-immune crosstalk in health and disease. Physiol Rev 2019;99(3):1325–80.
3. Irwin MR. Why sleep is important for health: a psychoneuroimmunology perspective. Annu Rev Psychol 2015;66:143–72.
4. Irwin MR, Opp MR. Sleep health: reciprocal regulation of sleep and innate immunity. Neuropsychopharmacology 2017;42(1):129–55.
5. Cappuccio FP, D'Elia L, Strazzullo P, et al. Quantity and quality of sleep and incidence of type 2 diabetes: a systematic review and meta-analysis. Diabetes Care 2010;33(2):414–20.

6. Trinder J, Waloszek J, Woods MJ, et al. Sleep and cardiovascular regulation. Pflugers Arch 2012; 463(1):161–8.

7. Walker MP. The role of sleep in cognition and emotion. Ann N Y Acad Sci 2009;1156:168–97.

8. Kryger M, Roth T, Dement W. Principles and practice of sleep medicine. 5th edition. New York: Saunders Elsevier; 2010.

9. de Zambotti M, Trinder J, Silvani A, et al. Dynamic coupling between the central and autonomic nervous systems during sleep: a review. Neurosci Biobehav Rev 2018;90:84–103.

10. Sadeh A. The role and validity of actigraphy in sleep medicine: an update. Sleep Med Rev 2011; 15(4):259–67.

11. de Zambotti M, Cellini N, Goldstone A, et al. Wearable sleep technology in clinical and research settings. Med Sci Sports Exerc 2019;51(7):1538–57.

12. Khosla S, Deak MC, Gault D, et al. Consumer sleep technology: an American Academy of Sleep Medicine position statement. J Clin Sleep Med 2018; 14(5):877–80.

13. Depner CM, Cheng PC, Devine JK, et al. Wearable technologies for developing sleep and circadian biomarkers: a summary of workshop discussions. Sleep 2019. [Epub ahead of print].

14. Consumer Technology Association. Performance Criteria and Testing Protocols for Features in Sleep Tracking Consumer Technology Devices and Applications (ANSI/CTA/NSF-2052.3). R11 Health & Fitness Technology Subcommittee; 2019.

15. Consumer Technology Association. Methodology of Measurements for Features in Sleep Tracking Consumer Technology Devices and Applications (ANSI/CTA/NSF-2052.2). R11 Health & Fitness Technology Subcommittee. 2017.

16. Consumer Technology Association. Definitions and Characteristics for Wearable Sleep Monitors (ANSI/CTA-NSF-2052.1). R11 Health & Fitness Technology Subcommittee. 2016.

17. Holter NJ. New method for heart studies. Science 1961;134(3486):1214–20.

18. Roebuck A, Monasterio V, Gederi E, et al. A review of signals used in sleep analysis. Physiol Meas 2013;35(1):R1–57.

19. Matar G, Lina J-M, Carrier J, et al. Unobtrusive sleep monitoring using cardiac, breathing and movements activities: an exhaustive review. IEEE Access 2018;6:45129–52.

20. Willemen T, Van Deun D, Verhaert V, et al. An evaluation of cardiorespiratory and movement features with respect to sleep-stage classification. IEEE J Biomed Health Inform 2014;18(2): 661–9.

21. Faust O, Razaghi H, Barika R, et al. A review of automated sleep stage scoring based on physiological signals for the new millennia.

Comput Methods Programs Biomed 2019;176: 81–91.

22. Herlan A, Ottenbacher J, Schneider J, et al. Electrodermal activity patterns in sleep stages and their utility for sleep versus wake classification. J Sleep Res 2019;28(2):e12694.

23. Danker-Hopfe H, Anderer P, Zeitlhofer J, et al. Inter-rater reliability for sleep scoring according to the Rechtschaffen & Kales and the new AASM standard. J Sleep Res 2009;18(1):74–84.

24. Radha M, Fonseca P, Moreau A, et al. Sleep stage classification from heart-rate variability using long short-term memory neural networks. Sci Rep 2019;9:14149.

25. Schäfer A, Vagedes J. How accurate is pulse rate variability as an estimate of heart rate variability? A review on studies comparing photoplethysmographic technology with an electrocardiogram. Int J Cardiol 2013;166(1):15–29.

26. Caspersen CJ, Powell KE, Christenson GM. Physical activity, exercise, and physical fitness: definitions and distinctions for health-related research. Public Health Rep 1985;100(2):126–31.

27. Chen KY, Bassett DR Jr. The technology of accelerometry-based activity monitors: current and future. Med Sci Sports Exerc 2005;37(11 Suppl):S490–500.

28. Reilly JJ, Penpraze V, Hislop J, et al. Objective measurement of physical activity and sedentary behaviour: review with new data. Arch Dis Child 2008;93(7):614–9.

29. Slater JA, Botsis T, Walsh J, et al. Assessing sleep using hip and wrist actigraphy. Sleep Biol Rhythms 2015;13(2):172–80.

30. Martin JL, Hakim AD. Wrist actigraphy. Chest 2011; 139(6):1514–27.

31. Van Hees VT, Sabia S, Anderson KN, et al. A novel, open access method to assess sleep duration using a wrist-worn accelerometer. PLoS One 2015; 10(11):e0142533.

32. Sadeh A, Sharkey KM, Carskadon MA. Activity-based sleep-wake identification: an empirical test of methodological issues. Sleep 1994;17(3):201–7.

33. Albinali F, Intille S, Haskell W, Rosenberger M. Using wearable activity type detection to improve physical activity energy expenditure estimation. In: proceedings from the Proceedings of the 12th ACM international conference on Ubiquitous computing. Copenhagen, September 26–29, 2010.

34. Middelkoop HA, Van Hilten BJ, Kramer CG, et al. Actigraphically recorded motor activity and immobility across sleep cycles and stages in healthy male subjects. J Sleep Res 1993;2(1):28–33.

35. Tryon WW. Issues of validity in actigraphic sleep assessment. Sleep 2004;27(1):158–65.

36. Morgenthaler T, Alessi C, Friedman L, et al. Practice parameters for the use of actigraphy in the

assessment of sleep and sleep disorders: an up-date for 2007. Sleep 2007;30(4):519–29.

37. van Hees VT, Sabia S, Jones SE, et al. Estimating sleep parameters using an accelerometer without sleep diary. Sci Rep 2018;8(1):12975.

38. Buysse DJ, Cheng Y, Germain A, et al. Night-to-night sleep variability in older adults with and without chronic insomnia. Sleep Med 2010;11(1): 56–64.

39. Natale V, Plazzi G, Martoni M. Actigraphy in the assessment of insomnia: a quantitative approach. Sleep 2009;32(6):767–71.

40. Cacioppo J, Tassinary L, Berntson G. Handbook of psychophysiology. 3rd edition. New York: Cambridge University Press; 2007.

41. Kligfield P, Gettes LS, Bailey JJ, et al. Recommendations for the standardization and interpretation of the electrocardiogram: part I: the electrocardiogram and its technology a scientific statement from the American Heart Association Electrocardiography and Arrhythmias Committee, Council on Clinical Cardiology; the American College of Cardiology Foundation; and the Heart Rhythm Society endorsed by the International Society for Computerized Electrocardiology. J Am Coll Cardiol 2007; 49(10):1109–27.

42. Parak J, Tarniceriu A, Renevey P, et al. Evaluation of the beat-to-beat detection accuracy of PulseOn wearable optical heart rate monitor. In: proceedings from the 2015 37th Annual International Conference of the IEEE Engineering in Medicine and Biology Society (EMBC). Milan, August 25–29, 2015.

43. Grossman P. The LifeShirt: a multi-function ambulatory system monitoring health, disease, and medical intervention in the real world. Stud Health Technol Inform 2004;108:133–41.

44. Laukkanen RM, Virtanen PK. Heart rate monitors: state of the art. J Sports Sci 1998;16(Suppl): S3–7.

45. Task Force of the European Society of Cardiology and the North American Society of Pacing and Electrophysiology. Heart rate variability: standards of measurement, physiological interpretation and clinical use. Task Force of the European Society of Cardiology and the North American Society of Pacing and Electrophysiology. Circulation 1996; 93(5):1043–65.

46. Benitez DS, Gaydecki P, Zaidi A, et al. A new QRS detection algorithm based on the Hilbert transform. In: Proceedings from the computers in cardiology 2000, vol. 27 (Cat. 00CH37163) Cambridge, September 24–27, 2000.

47. Ruha A, Sallinen S, Nissila S. A real-time microprocessor QRS detector system with a 1-ms timing accuracy for the measurement of ambulatory HRV. IEEE Trans Biomed Eng 1997;44(3):159–67.

48. Berntson GG, Quigley KS, Jang JF, et al. An approach to artifact identification: application to heart period data. Psychophysiology 1990;27(5): 586–98.

49. Kaufmann T, Sutterlin S, Schulz SM, et al. ARTiiFACT: a tool for heart rate artifact processing and heart rate variability analysis. Behav Res Methods 2011;43(4):1161–70.

50. Laborde S, Mosley E, Thayer JF. Heart rate variability and cardiac vagal tone in psychophysiological research - Recommendations for experiment planning, data analysis, and data reporting. Front Psychol 2017;8:213.

51. Fonseca P, Long X, Radha M, et al. Sleep stage classification with ECG and respiratory effort. Physiol Meas 2015;36(10):2027–40.

52. Allen J. Photoplethysmography and its application in clinical physiological measurement. Physiol Meas 2007;28(3):R1–39.

53. Elgendi M. On the analysis of fingertip photoplethysmogram signals. Curr Cardiol Rev 2012;8(1): 14–25.

54. Sun Y, Thakor N. Photoplethysmography revisited: from contact to noncontact, from point to imaging. IEEE Trans Biomed Eng 2016;63(3): 463–77.

55. Van de Louw A, Cracco C, Cerf C, et al. Accuracy of pulse oximetry in the intensive care unit. Intensive Care Med 2001;27(10):1606–13.

56. Henriksen A, Mikalsen MH, Woldaregay AZ, et al. Using fitness trackers and smartwatches to measure physical activity in research: analysis of consumer wrist-worn wearables. J Med Internet Res 2018;20(3):e110.

57. Akar SA, Kara S, Latifoğlu F, et al. Spectral analysis of photoplethysmographic signals: the importance of preprocessing. Biomed Signal Process Control 2013;8(1):16–22.

58. Spierer DK, Rosen Z, Litman LL, et al. Validation of photoplethysmography as a method to detect heart rate during rest and exercise. J Med Eng Technol 2015;39(5):264–71.

59. Maeda Y, Sekine M, Tamura T. Relationship between measurement site and motion artifacts in wearable reflected photoplethysmography. J Med Syst 2011;35(5):969–76.

60. Shin H. Ambient temperature effect on pulse rate variability as an alternative to heart rate variability in young adult. J Clin Monit Comput 2016;30(6):939–48.

61. Beattie Z, Pantelopoulos A, Ghoreyshi A, et al. 0068 estimation of sleep stages using cardiac and accelerometer data from a wrist-worn device. Sleep 2017;40(suppl_1):A26.

62. Fonseca P, Weysen T, Goelema MS, et al. Validation of photoplethysmography-based sleep staging compared with polysomnography in healthy middle-aged adults. Sleep 2017;40(7).

63. Uçar MK, Bozkurt MR, Bilgin C, et al. Automatic sleep staging in obstructive sleep apnea patients using photoplethysmography, heart rate variability signal and machine learning techniques. Neural Comput Appl 2018;29(8):1–16.

64. Al-Khalidi FQ, Saatchi R, Burke D, et al. Respiration rate monitoring methods: a review. Pediatr Pulmonol 2011;46(6):523–9.

65. Wientjes CJ. Respiration in psychophysiology: methods and applications. Biol Psychol 1992; 34(2–3):179–203.

66. Charlton PH, Bonnici T, Tarassenko L, et al. An assessment of algorithms to estimate respiratory rate from the electrocardiogram and photoplethysmogram. Physiol Meas 2016;37(4): 610–26.

67. Meredith DJ, Clifton D, Charlton P, et al. Photoplethysmographic derivation of respiratory rate: a review of relevant physiology. J Med Eng Technol 2012;36(1):1–7.

68. Long X, Yang J, Weysen T, et al. Measuring dissimilarity between respiratory effort signals based on uniform scaling for sleep staging. Physiol Meas 2014;35(12):2529.

69. Netzer N, Eliasson AH, Netzer C, et al. Overnight pulse oximetry for sleep-disordered breathing in adults: a review. Chest 2001;120(2):625–33.

70. Lim CL, Byrne C, Lee JK. Human thermoregulation and measurement of body temperature in exercise and clinical settings. Ann Acad Med Singapore 2008;37(4):347–53.

71. Romanovsky AA. Thermoregulation: some concepts have changed. Functional architecture of the thermoregulatory system. Am J Physiol Regul Integr Comp Physiol 2007;292(1):R37–46.

72. Van Someren EJ. Mechanisms and functions of coupling between sleep and temperature rhythms. Prog Brain Res 2006;153:309–24.

73. Schey BM, Williams DY, Bucknall T. Skin temperature and core-peripheral temperature gradient as markers of hemodynamic status in critically ill patients: a review. Heart Lung 2010;39(1):27–40.

74. Podtaev S, Morozov M, Frick P. Wavelet-based correlations of skin temperature and blood flow oscillations. Cardiovasc Eng 2008;8(3):185–9.

75. Shusterman V, Anderson KP, Barnea O. Spontaneous skin temperature oscillations in normal human subjects. Am J Physiol 1997;273(3 Pt 2): R1173–81.

76. Stoker MR. Measuring temperature. Anaesth Intensive Care Med 2005;6(6):194–8.

77. van Marken Lichtenbelt WD, Daanen HA, Wouters L, et al. Evaluation of wireless determination of skin temperature using iButtons. Physiol Behav 2006;88(4–5):489–97.

78. Van Someren EJ. More than a marker: interaction between the circadian regulation of temperature and sleep, age-related changes, and treatment possibilities. Chronobiol Int 2000;17(3):313–54.

79. Keränen K, Mäkinen J-T, Korhonen P, et al. Infrared temperature sensor system for mobile devices. Sens Actuators A Phys 2010;158(1):161–7.

80. Choi JK, Miki K, Sagawa S, et al. Evaluation of mean skin temperature formulas by infrared thermography. Int J Biometeorol 1997;41(2):68–75.

81. Nielsen R, Nielsen B. Measurement of mean skin temperature of clothed persons in cool environments. Eur J Appl Physiol Occup Physiol 1984; 53(3):231–6.

82. Oliver SJ, Costa RJ, Laing SJ, et al. One night of sleep deprivation decreases treadmill endurance performance. Eur J Appl Physiol 2009;107(2):155–61.

83. Kräuchi K, Cajochen C, Werth E, et al. Physiology: warm feet promote the rapid onset of sleep. Nature 1999;401(6748):36.

84. Sarabia JA, Rol MA, Mendiola P, et al. Circadian rhythm of wrist temperature in normal-living subjects A candidate of new index of the circadian system. Physiol Behav 2008;95(4):570–80.

85. Zhou SM, Hill RA, Morgan K, et al. Classification of accelerometer wear and non-wear events in seconds for monitoring free-living physical activity. BMJ Open 2015;5(5):e007447.

86. Boucsein W. Electrodermal activity. Boston: Springer Science & Business Media; 2012.

87. Critchley HD. Electrodermal responses: what happens in the brain. Neuroscientist 2002;8(2):132–42.

88. Fowles DC, Christie MJ, Edelberg R, et al. Committee report. Publication recommendations for electrodermal measurements. Psychophysiology 1981;18(3):232–9.

89. Nordbotten B, Tronstad C, Martinsen Ø, et al. Estimation of skin conductance at low frequencies using measurements at higher frequencies for EDA applications. Physiological measurement 2014; 35(6):1011–8.

90. Freedman LW, Scerbo AS, Dawson ME, et al. The relationship of sweat gland count to electrodermal activity. Psychophysiology 1994;31(2):196–200.

91. Poh MZ, Loddenkemper T, Reinsberger C, et al. Convulsive seizure detection using a wrist-worn electrodermal activity and accelerometry biosensor. Epilepsia 2012;53(5):e93–7.

92. Lee B-G, Chung W-Y. Wearable glove-type driver stress detection using a motion sensor. IEEE Trans Intell Transport Syst 2016;18(7):1835–44.

93. Kappeler-Setz C, Gravenhorst F, Schumm J, et al. Towards long term monitoring of electrodermal activity in daily life. Pers Ubiquitous Comput 2013; 17(2):261–71.

94. Bach DR. A head-to-head comparison of SCRalyze and Ledalab, two model-based methods for skin conductance analysis. Biol Psychol 2014;103: 63–8.

95. Benedek M, Kaernbach C. A continuous measure of phasic electrodermal activity. J Neurosci Methods 2010;190(1):80–91.

96. Boucsein W, Fowles DC, Grimnes S, et al. Publication recommendations for electrodermal measurements. Psychophysiology 2012;49(8):1017–34.

97. van Dooren M, de Vries JJ, Janssen JH. Emotional sweating across the body: comparing 16 different skin conductance measurement locations. Physiol Behav 2012;106(2):298–304.

98. Koumans AJ, Tursky B, Solomon P. Electrodermal levels and fluctuations during normal sleep. Psychophysiology 1968;5(3):300–6.

99. Sano A, Picard RW, Stickgold R. Quantitative analysis of wrist electrodermal activity during sleep. Int J Psychophysiol 2014;94(3):382–9.

100. Weise S, Ong J, Tesler NA, et al. Worried sleep: 24-h monitoring in high and low worriers. Biol Psychol 2013;94(1):61–70.

101. Onorati F, Regalia G, Caborni C, et al. Multicenter clinical assessment of improved wearable multi-modal convulsive seizure detectors. Epilepsia 2017;58(11):1870–9.

102. de Zambotti M, Colrain IM, Javitz HS, et al. Magnitude of the impact of hot flashes on sleep in perimenopausal women. Fertil Steril 2014;102(6):1708–15.e1.

103. Baker F, Forouzanfar M, Goldstone A, et al. Changes in heart rate and blood pressure across nocturnal hot flashes associated with or without arousal from sleep. Sleep 2019;42(11) [pii:zsz175].

104. Roenneberg T, Kuehnle T, Juda M, et al. Epidemiology of the human circadian clock. Sleep Med Rev 2007;11(6):429–38.

105. Reppert SM, Weaver DR. Coordination of circadian timing in mammals. Nature 2002;418(6901):935–41.

106. Faulkner SM, Bee PE, Meyer N, et al. Light therapies to improve sleep in intrinsic circadian rhythm sleep disorders and neuro-psychiatric illness: a systematic review and meta-analysis. Sleep Med Rev 2019;46:108–23.

107. Hunter CM, Figueiro MG. Measuring light at night and melatonin levels in shift workers: a review of the literature. Biol Res Nurs 2017;19(4):365–74.

108. Kozaki T, Koga S, Toda N, et al. Effects of short wavelength control in polychromatic light sources on nocturnal melatonin secretion. Neurosci Lett 2008;439(3):256–9.

109. Rea MS, Figueiro MG, Bullough JD. Circadian photobiology: an emerging framework for lighting practice and research. Light Res Technol 2002;34(3):177–87.

110. Miller D, Bierman A, Figueiro M, et al. Ecological measurements of light exposure, activity, and circadian disruption. Light Res Technol 2010;42(3):271–84.

111. Landis EG, Yang V, Brown DM, et al. Dim light exposure and myopia in children. Invest Ophthalmol Vis Sci 2018;59(12):4804–11.

112. Kamisalic A, Fister I Jr, Turkanovic M, et al. Sensors and functionalities of non-invasive wrist-wearable devices: a review. Sensors (Basel) 2018;18(6):1714.

113. Borazio M, Van Laerhoven K. Combining wearable and environmental sensing into an unobtrusive tool for long-term sleep studies. In: Proceedings from the Proceedings of the 2nd ACM SIGHIT International Health Informatics Symposium. Miami, January 28 - 30, 2012.

114. Rea MS, Bierman A, Figueiro MG, et al. A new approach to understanding the impact of circadian disruption on human health. J Circadian Rhythms 2008;6(1):7.

115. Bandodkar AJ, Wang J. Non-invasive wearable electrochemical sensors: a review. Trends Biotechnol 2014;32(7):363–71.

116. Peake JM, Kerr G, Sullivan JP. A critical review of consumer wearables, mobile applications, and equipment for providing biofeedback, monitoring stress, and sleep in physically active populations. Front Physiol 2018;9:743.

117. Fahrenberg J, Myrtek M, Pawlik K, et al. Ambulatory assessment–Monitoring behavior in daily life settings: a behavioral-scientific challenge for psychology. Eur J Psychol Assess 2007;23(4):206.

118. Jeng P, Wang L-C. Stream data analysis of body sensors for sleep posture monitoring: an automatic labelling approach. In: proceedings from the 2017 26th Wireless and Optical Communication Conference (WOCC). Newark, April 7–8, 2017.

119. de Zambotti M, Baker F, Willoughby A, et al. Measures of sleep and cardiac functioning during sleep using a multi-sensory commercially-available wristband in adolescents. Physiol Behav 2016;158:143–9.

120. Haghayegh S, Khoshnevis S, Smolensky MH, et al. Accuracy of PurePulse photoplethysmography technology of Fitbit charge 2 for assessment of heart rate during sleep. Chronobiol Int 2019;36(7):927–33.

121. Iber C, Ancoli-Israel S, Chesson A, et al. The AASM manual for the scoring of sleep and associated events: rules, terminology, and technical specification. 1st edition. Westchester (IL): American Academy of Sleep Medicine; 2007.

122. de Zambotti M, Claudatos S, Inkelis S, et al. Evaluation of a consumer fitness-tracking device to assess sleep in adults. Chronobiol Int 2015;32(7):1024–8.

123. de Zambotti M, Goldstone A, Claudatos S, et al. A validation study of Fitbit charge 2 compared with polysomnography in adults. Chronobiol Int 2018;35(4):465–76.

124. Ameen M, Cheung L, Hauser T, et al. About the accuracy and problems of consumer devices in the assessment of sleep. Sensors (Basel) 2019; 19(19) [pii:E4160].

125. Cook JD, Prairie ML, Plante DT. Utility of the Fitbit Flex to evaluate sleep in major depressive disorder: a comparison against polysomnography and wrist-worn actigraphy. J Affect Disord 2017;217: 299–305.

126. Kahawage P, Jumabhoy R, Hamill K, et al. Validity, potential clinical utility, and comparison of consumer and research-grade activity trackers in insomnia disorder I: in-lab validation against polysomnography. J Sleep Res 2019. [Epub ahead of print].

127. Cook JD, Prairie ML, Plante DT. Ability of the multisensory jawbone UP3 to quantify and classify sleep in patients with suspected central disorders of hypersomnolence: a comparison against polysomnography and actigraphy. J Clin Sleep Med 2018;14(5):841–8.

128. Cook JD, Eftekari SC, Dallmann E, et al. Ability of the Fitbit Alta HR to quantify and classify sleep in patients with suspected central disorders of hypersomnolence: a comparison against polysomnography. J Sleep Res 2019;28(4):e12789.

129. de Zambotti M, Rosas L, Colrain IM, et al. The sleep of the ring: comparison of the OURA sleep tracker against polysomnography. Behav Sleep Med 2017;21:1–15.

130. Mantua J, Gravel N, Spencer RM. Reliability of sleep measures from four personal health monitoring devices compared to research-based actigraphy and polysomnography. Sensors (Basel) 2016;16(5):646.

131. Meltzer LJ, Walsh CM, Peightal AA. Comparison of actigraphy immobility rules with polysomnographic sleep onset latency in children and adolescents. Sleep Breath 2015;19(4):1415–23.

132. Toon E, Davey M, Hollis S, et al. Comparison of commercial wrist-based and smartphone accelerometers, actigraphy, and PSG in a clinical cohort of children and adolescents. J Clin Sleep Med 2015;12(3):343–50.

133. Pesonen AK, Kuula L. The validity of a new consumer-targeted wrist device in sleep measurement: an overnight comparison against polysomnography in children and adolescents. J Clin Sleep Med 2018;14(4):585–91.

134. de Zambotti M, Baker FC, Colrain IM. Validation of sleep-tracking technology compared with polysomnography in adolescents. Sleep 2015;38(9):1461–8.

135. Danzig R, Wang M, Shah A, et al. The wrist is not the brain: estimation of sleep by clinical and consumer wearable actigraphy devices is impacted by multiple patient- and device-specific factors. J Sleep Res 2019. [Epub ahead of print].

136. Meltzer LJ, Hiruma LS, Avis K, et al. Comparison of a commercial accelerometer with polysomnography and actigraphy in children and adolescents. Sleep 2015;38(8):1323–30.

137. Kang SG, Kang JM, Ko KP, et al. Validity of a commercial wearable sleep tracker in adult insomnia disorder patients and good sleepers. J Psychosom Res 2017;97:38–44.

138. Maskevich S, Jumabhoy R, Dao PDM, et al. Pilot validation of ambulatory activity monitors for sleep measurement in huntington's disease gene carriers. J Huntingtons Dis 2017;6(3):249–53.

139. Dunn J, Runge R, Snyder M. Wearables and the medical revolution. Per Med 2018;15(5):429–48.

140. Bertz JW, Epstein DH, Preston KL. Combining ecological momentary assessment with objective, ambulatory measures of behavior and physiology in substance-use research. Addict Behav 2018; 83:5–17.

141. Colombo D, Fernandez-Alvarez J, Patane A, et al. Current state and future directions of technology-based ecological momentary assessment and intervention for major depressive disorder: a systematic review. J Clin Med 2019;8(4):465.

142. Seppala J, De Vita I, Jamsa T, et al. Mobile phone and wearable sensor-based mHealth approaches for psychiatric disorders and symptoms: systematic review. JMIR Ment Health 2019;6(2):e9819.

143. Shiffman S, Stone AA, Hufford MR. Ecological momentary assessment. Annu Rev Clin Psychol 2008;4:1–32.

144. Jain SH, Powers BW, Hawkins JB, et al. The digital phenotype. Nat Biotechnol 2015;33(5):462–3.

145. Hong YJ, Jeong H, Cho KW, et al. Wearable and implantable devices for cardiovascular healthcare: from monitoring to therapy based on flexible and stretchable electronics. Adv Funct Mater 2019; 29(19):1808247.

146. Nagai M, Hoshide S, Kario K. Sleep duration as a risk factor for cardiovascular disease-a review of the recent literature. Curr Cardiol Rev 2010;6(1): 54–61.

147. Cooney MT, Vartiainen E, Laatikainen T, et al. Elevated resting heart rate is an independent risk factor for cardiovascular disease in healthy men and women. Am Heart J 2010;159(4):612–9.e3.

148. Teo JX, Davila S, Yang C, et al. Digital phenotyping by consumer wearables identifies sleep-associated markers of cardiovascular disease risk and biological aging. Commun Biol 2019;2:361.

149. McDonald L, Mehmud F, Ramagopalan SV. Sleep and BMI: do (Fitbit) bands aid? F1000Res 2018; 7:511.

150. Xu X, Conomos MP, Manor O, et al. Habitual sleep duration and sleep duration variation are independently associated with body mass index. Int J Obes (Lond) 2018;42(4):794–800.

151. Turel O, Romashkin A, Morrison KM. Health outcomes of information system use lifestyles among adolescents: videogame addiction, sleep curtailment and cardio-metabolic deficiencies. PLoS One 2016;11(5):e0154764.

152. Ballinger B, Hsieh J, Singh A, et al. DeepHeart: semi-supervised sequence learning for cardiovascular risk prediction. In: Proceedings from the Thirty-Second AAAI Conference on Artificial Intelligence. New Orleans, February 2–7, 2018.

153. Tison GH, Sanchez JM, Ballinger B, et al. Passive detection of atrial fibrillation using a commercially available smartwatch. JAMA Cardiol 2018;3(5):409–16.

154. Cho C-H, Lee T, Kim M-G, et al. Mood prediction of patients with mood disorders by machine learning using passive digital phenotypes based on the circadian rhythm: prospective observational cohort study. J Med Internet Res 2019;21(4):e11029.

155. Bian J, Guo Y, Xie M, et al. Exploring the association between self-reported asthma impact and Fitbit-derived sleep quality and physical activity measures in adolescents. JMIR Mhealth Uhealth 2017;5(7):e105.

156. Weatherall J, Paprocki Y, Meyer TM, et al. Sleep tracking and exercise in patients with type 2 diabetes mellitus (step-D): pilot study to determine correlations between fitbit data and patient-reported outcomes. JMIR Mhealth Uhealth 2018;6(6):e131.

157. Dunn J, Huebner E, Liu S, et al. Using consumer-grade wearables and novel measures of sleep and activity to analyze changes in behavioral health during an 8-month simulated Mars mission. Comput Ind 2017;92:32–42.

158. Kang SG, Kang JM, Cho SJ, et al. Cognitive behavioral therapy using a mobile application synchronizable with wearable devices for insomnia treatment: a pilot study. J Clin Sleep Med 2017;13(4):633–40.

159. Gruwez A, Bruyneel AV, Bruyneel M. The validity of two commercially-available sleep trackers and actigraphy for assessment of sleep parameters in obstructive sleep apnea patients. PLoS One 2019;14(1):e0210569.

160. Moreno-Pino F, Porras-Segovia A, López-Esteban P, et al. Validation of Fitbit charge 2 and Fitbit Alta HR against polysomnography for assessing sleep in adults with obstructive sleep apnea. J Clin Sleep Med 2019;15(11):1645–53.

161. Rosa TD, Zitser J, Capasso R. Consumer technology for sleep-disordered breathing: a review of the landscape. Curr Otorhinolaryngol Rep 2019;7(1):18–26.

162. Camci B, Ersoy C, Kaynak H. Abnormal respiratory event detection in sleep: a prescreening system with smart wearables. J Biomed Inform 2019;95:103218.

163. Le TQ, Cheng C, Sangasoongsong A, et al. Wireless wearable multisensory suite and real-time prediction of obstructive sleep apnea episodes. IEEE J Transl Eng Health Med 2013;1:2700109.

164. Crowley O, Pugliese L, Kachnowski S. The impact of wearable device enabled health initiative on physical activity and sleep. Cureus 2016;8(10):e825.

165. Melton BF, Buman MP, Vogel RL, et al. Wearable devices to improve physical activity and sleep. J Black Stud 2016;47(6):610–25.

166. Luik AI, Machado PF, Espie CA. Delivering digital cognitive behavioral therapy for insomnia at scale: does using a wearable device to estimate sleep influence therapy? NPJ Digit Med 2018;1(1):3.

167. Dunican IC, Martin DT, Halson SL, et al. The effects of the removal of electronic devices for 48 hours on sleep in elite judo athletes. J Strength Cond Res 2017;31(10):2832–9.

168. Rondanelli M, Opizzi A, Monteferrario F, et al. The effect of melatonin, magnesium, and zinc on primary insomnia in long-term care facility residents in Italy: a double-blind, placebo-controlled clinical trial. J Am Geriatr Soc 2011;59(1):82–90.

169. Zhang Z, Cajochen C, Khatami R. Social jetlag and chronotypes in the Chinese population: analysis of data recorded by wearable devices. J Med Internet Res 2019;21(6):e13482.

170. Dewald JF, Meijer AM, Oort FJ, et al. The influence of sleep quality, sleep duration and sleepiness on school performance in children and adolescents: a meta-analytic review. Sleep Med Rev 2010;14(3):179–89.

171. Phillips AJK, Clerx WM, O'Brien CS, et al. Irregular sleep/wake patterns are associated with poorer academic performance and delayed circadian and sleep/wake timing. Sci Rep 2017;7(1):3216.

172. Chu HC, Liu YM, Kuo FR. A mobile sleep-management learning system for improving students' sleeping habits by integrating a self-regulated learning strategy: randomized controlled trial. JMIR Mhealth Uhealth 2018;6(10):e11557.

173. Sano A, Phillips AJ, Amy ZY, et al. Recognizing academic performance, sleep quality, stress level, and mental health using personality traits, wearable sensors and mobile phones. In: Proceedings from the 2015 IEEE 12th International Conference on Wearable and Implantable Body Sensor Networks (BSN). Cambridge, June 9–12, 2015.

174. Wang R, Chen F, Chen Z, et al. StudentLife: assessing mental health, academic performance and behavioral trends of college students using smartphones. In: Proceedings from the Proceedings of the 2014 ACM international joint conference

on pervasive and ubiquitous computing. Seattle, September 13–17, 2014.

175. Thun E, Bjorvatn B, Flo E, et al. Sleep, circadian rhythms, and athletic performance. Sleep Med Rev 2015;23:1–9.

176. Fullagar HH, Duffield R, Skorski S, et al. Sleep and recovery in team sport: current sleep-related issues facing professional team-sport athletes. Int J Sports Physiol Perform 2015;10(8):950–7.

177. Simpson NS, Gibbs EL, Matheson GO. Optimizing sleep to maximize performance: implications and recommendations for elite athletes. Scand J Med Sci Sports 2017;27(3):266–74.

178. Halson SL, Peake JM, Sullivan JP. Wearable technology for athletes: information overload and pseudoscience? Int J Sports Physiol Perform 2016; 11(6):705–6.

179. Sargent C, Lastella M, Romyn G, et al. How well does a commercially available wearable device measure sleep in young athletes? Chronobiol Int 2018;35(6):754–8.

180. Plews DJ, Laursen PB, Stanley J, et al. Training adaptation and heart rate variability in elite endurance athletes: opening the door to effective monitoring. Sports Med 2013;43(9):773–81.

181. Altini M, Van Hoof C, Amft O. Relation between estimated cardiorespiratory fitness and running performance in free-living: an analysis of HRV4Training data. In: Proceedings from the 2017 IEEE EMBS International Conference on Biomedical & Health Informatics (BHI). Orlando, February 16–19, 2017.

182. Linton SJ, Kecklund G, Franklin KA, et al. The effect of the work environment on future sleep disturbances: a systematic review. Sleep Med Rev 2015;23:10–9.

183. Törnroos M, Hakulinen C, Hintsanen M, et al. Reciprocal relationships between psychosocial work characteristics and sleep problems: a two-wave study. Work Stress 2017;31(1):63–81.

184. Sonnentag S, Binnewies C, Mojza EJ. "Did you have a nice evening?" A day-level study on recovery experiences, sleep, and affect. J Appl Psychol 2008;93(3):674.

185. Demerouti E, Bakker A, Geurts S, et al. Daily recovery from work-related effort during non-work time. In: Sonnentag S, Perrewé P, Ganster D, editors. Current Perspectives on Job-Stress Recovery (Research in Occupational Stress and Well Being, Vol. 7). Bingley: Emerald Group Publishing Limited; 2009. p. 85–123.

186. Binnewies C, Sonnentag S, Mojza EJ. Daily performance at work: feeling recovered in the morning as a predictor of day-level job performance. J Organ Behav 2009;30(1):67–93.

187. Kompier M. Assessing the psychosocial work environment–"Subjective" versus "objective" measurement. Scand J Work Environ Health 2005;31(6):405–8.

188. Semmer N, Grebner S, Elfering A. BEYOND SELF-REPORT: USING OBSERVATIONAL, PHYSIOLOGICAL, AND SITUATION-BASED MEASURES IN RESEARCH ON OCCUPATIONAL STRESS. In: Perrewe P, Ganster D, editors. Emotional and Physiological Processes and Positive Intervention Strategies (Research in Occupational Stress and Well Being, Vol. 3). Bingley: Emerald Group Publishing Limited; 2003. p. 205–63.

189. Yassierli Y, Sari R, Muslim K. Evaluating smartwatch-based sleep quality indicators of fitness to work. Int J Tech 2017;8(2):329.

190. Mirjafari S, Masaba K, Grover T, et al. Differentiating higher and lower job performers in the workplace using mobile sensing. Proc ACM Interact Mob Wearable Ubiquitous Technol 2019;3(2):37.

191. Ferguson SA, Appleton SL, Reynolds AC, et al. Making errors at work due to sleepiness or sleep problems is not confined to non-standard work hours: results of the 2016 Sleep Health Foundation national survey. Chronobiol Int 2019;36(6):758–69.

192. Folkard S, Lombardi DA, Tucker PT. Shiftwork: safety, sleepiness and sleep. Ind Health 2005; 43(1):20–3.

193. Horne J, Reyner L. Sleep-related vehicle accidents: some guides for road safety policies. Transp Res Part F Traffic Psychol Behav 2001;4(1):63–74.

194. Mollicone D, Kan K, Mott C, et al. Predicting performance and safety based on driver fatigue. Accid Anal Prev 2019;126:142–5.

195. Al-Libawy H, Al-Ataby A, Al-Nuaimy W, et al. Estimation of driver alertness using low-cost wearable devices. In: Proceedings from the 2015 IEEE Jordan Conference on Applied Electrical Engineering and Computing Technologies (AEECT). Amman, November 3–5, 2015.

196. Al-Libawy H, Al-Ataby A, Al-Nuaimy W, et al. HRV-based operator fatigue analysis and classification using wearable sensors. In: Proceedings from the 2016 13th International Multi-Conference on Systems, Signals & Devices (SSD). Leipzig, March 21–24, 2016.

197. Goel B, Dey AK, Bharti P, et al. Detecting distracted driving using a wrist-worn wearable. In: proceedings from the 2018 IEEE International Conference on Pervasive Computing and Communications Workshops (PerCom Workshops). Athens, March 19–23, 2018.

198. Zheng W-L, Gao K, Li G, et al. Vigilance estimation using a wearable EOG device in real driving environment. IEEE Transactions on Intelligent Transportation Systems; 2019. p. 1–15.

You Snooze, You Win? An Ecological Dynamics Framework Approach to Understanding the Relationships Between Sleep and Sensorimotor Performance in Sport

Alice D. LaGoy, MS[a,b], Fabio Ferrarelli, MD, PhD[b],
Aaron M. Sinnott, MS, ATC[a], Shawn R. Eagle, PhD, ATC, CSCS[c],
Caleb D. Johnson, PhD[d], Christopher Connaboy, PhD[a,*]

KEYWORDS

• Visuomotor • Affordance • Perception-action coupling • Sleep • Spindles • Slow wave sleep

KEY POINTS

- Sensorimotor performance refers to the ability of an individual to effectively couple sensory information and motor output in a dynamic and continuous fashion.
- Sleep may enhance sensorimotor performance through synaptic remodeling of brain regions active during task performance.
- Specific sleep features, namely spindles, slow wave activity, and potentially rapid eye movement sleep, correspond to sensorimotor enhancement.
- Future work is needed to understand whether targeted generation of sleep features can improve performance.

INTRODUCTION

To be at the top of their sport, athletes must operate at a high level and recover quickly after demanding training sessions and competitions. One perceived barrier to optimal performance in athletes is poor sleep hygiene.[1,2] Many athletes have to endure demanding travel schedules that may lead to circadian misalignment.[3,4] Furthermore, early morning practices and late-night games can influence sleep duration[2,5] whereas precompetition anxiety and postcompetition muscle soreness may compromise sleep quality.[6] These interruptions to healthy sleep may compromise performance, impair recovery, and increase risk of injury.[2,7]

Prior sleep has an impact on next-day function by influencing cognitive capabilities[8] and physical performance[7] but optimal sports performance also requires timely and accurate sensorimotor function.[9–11] Worse sports performance, such as

[a] Department of Sports Medicine and Nutrition, University of Pittsburgh, 3860 South Water Street, Pittsburgh, PA 15203, USA; [b] Department of Psychiatry, University of Pittsburgh School of Medicine, 3501 Forbes Avenue, Suite 456, Pittsburgh, PA 15213, USA; [c] Rooney Sports Medicine Concussion Program, Department of Orthopaedic Surgery, University of Pittsburgh Medical Center, University of Pittsburgh School of Medicine, 3850 South Water Street, Pittsburgh, PA 15203, USA; [d] Department of Physical Medicine and Rehabilitation, Harvard Medical School, 1575 Cambridge Street, Cambridge, MA 02138, USA
* Corresponding author. Neuromuscular Research Laboratory, Department of Sports Medicine and Nutrition, 3860 South Water Street, Pittsburgh, PA 15203.
E-mail address: connaboy@pitt.edu

Sleep Med Clin 15 (2020) 31–39
https://doi.org/10.1016/j.jsmc.2019.11.001
1556-407X/20/© 2019 Elsevier Inc. All rights reserved.

lower on-base percentage in baseball and lower shooting accuracy in hockey, have been associated with poor sensorimotor performance.[9–11] In turn, poor sleep has been associated with deficits in motor skill–specific learning and plasticity, key components of sensorimotor performance for athletes.[12–14] Sleep-related changes in sensorimotor performance may be attributed to specific features of sleep, such as slow waves[12,15,16] and spindles.[17–19]

The ecological dynamics framework describes the direct perception of sensory information and continuous coupling of this information with motor behaviors, providing an accurate description of sensorimotor function.[20–22] Through direct perception, an individual initiates appropriate motor responses based on perceptions of the surrounding environment without the need to cognitively process this information; perceptual information is inherently meaningful.[23] The coupling between perception and action described within the framework is essential to the execution of actions that require adaptation to dynamic changes in the environment, such as fielding a baseball that takes an unexpected bounce.[22,24] Sleep influences sensorimotor performance by altering different aspects of sensorimotor function, including perception-action coupling.[25,26] This review defines sensorimotor performance from an ecological dynamics framework, describes the interaction between sleep and sensorimotor performance by examining the general influence of sleep as well as the influence of more granular sleep features, and, finally, discusses directions for future research encompassing the ecological dynamics framework.

DEFINING SENSORIMOTOR PERFORMANCE AND IMPLICATIONS FOR BEHAVIORAL INJURY RISK

Examining sensorimotor performance from an ecological perspective emphasizes movement behavior as a coupling between the sensory and motor systems, which operate in a cooperative and integrated fashion to increase the likelihood of successful and appropriate action.[22] Individuals directly perceive relevant sensory information from the environment and modulate their actions according to the continuous updating of this sensory information.[20,21] Importantly, an individual must perceive how characteristics of the environment influence the ability to act within the environment. Affordances are the opportunities for action created by the interaction between characteristics of the environment and capabilities of the individual.[20,22,23] Affordances change across time as

characteristics of the environment and capabilities of the individual change. For example, increasing fatigue throughout a game can compromise the action capabilities of an athlete. Athletes must be attuned to how changes in their action capabilities influence action boundaries (ie, the limits of possible actions) and must adapt their actions by recalibrating to this change in their action capabilities.[23,27] Furthermore, the ability of individuals to perceive affordances changes when they experience a systemic perturbation, such as under conditions of sleep deprivation[25,26] or when recovering from a concussion.[28,29] If individuals are not attuned to changes in affordances, they may attempt to complete actions that are not possible. Furthermore, if they are unable to execute/modulate actions in a timely manner, they may attempt to complete an action when the behavior is no longer afforded. Therefore, systemic perturbations, such as sleep deprivation, not only may compromise the action capabilities of athletes but also may contribute to inaccurate affordance perception, thereby compromising sensorimotor function and increasing behavioral risk.[30]

For example, a football player who misjudges the ability to run between 2 defenders is more likely to be tackled than one who perceives the position and trajectories of the defenders and adjusts the path accordingly.[28] Worse performance on a laboratory-based sensorimotor battery was associated with increased head impact severity in football players, suggesting individuals with worse sensorimotor capabilities placed themselves in injurious position, whereas individuals with better sensorimotor capabilities could adjust their actions to minimize such impacts.[9] Importantly, traditional reaction time measures did not find similar relationships between performance and head impacts, suggesting that the relationship was specific to sensorimotor performance and not simply a factor of vigilance and reaction time.[9] If sleep is related to sensorimotor performance, compromised sleep during the season may have an impact on the injury risk of athletes in addition to compromising overall performance. This may be especially important for athletes who participate in tournament-style competitions, such as swimmers, hockey players, and rugby sevens players, where sleep curtailment may be more prevalent.

Sports involve dynamically changing environments; individuals must be attuned to changes within these environments and must modulate their actions according to continuously updating perceptual information. As such, better sport-specific sensorimotor performance in expert performers may be related to an improved ability to attune to relevant perceptual information, which allows for more effective perception-action coupling.[31–33] Improved attunement and performance in expert baseball and cricket batters are related to more efficient gaze strategies that use anticipatory saccades to track ball flight and more stable head-tracking strategies.[24,34,35] Furthermore, expert performers often attune to relevant stimuli, such as kinematics of opponents, in a more timely and anticipatory fashion, which allows them to initiate motor responses earlier and to modulate responses throughout the action.[34,36] Increased movement variability has been observed early in motor responses of expert performers, suggesting that they are able to continuously modulate their motor responses based on updated perceptual information.[24,37] Importantly, improved performance is observed when athletes are able to complete a motor response compared with when they are asked to make an explicit judgment about what their response would be. This suggests that active engagement with and exploration of the environment are needed for optimal sensorimotor function.[31] In that way, the relationship between perception and action is reciprocal; perception drives action and action drives perception.[20,23]

Because sleep has been shown to effect the ability to track visual stimuli, sleep may play a vital role in perceptual aspects of sensorimotor function and the successful execution of sporting performances.[38] During the night after practice of sensorimotor tasks, changes in brain activity in task-specific (eg, visual or motor) regions of the brain suggest that sleep may play a role across more aspects of sensorimotor function.[12,39,40] Within the visual system, 2 distinct streams contribute to different aspects of affordance-based performance and sensorimotor function.[41–43] The ventral stream connects the visual cortex to the inferotemporal cortex and is responsible for identifying and perceiving characteristics of objects essential to affordance perception.[41,42] The dorsal stream connects the primary visual cortex to the posterior parietal cortex and is responsible for the quick modulation of action in response to visual information.[42] As such, the ventral stream is often said to be responsible for "vision for perception" whereas the dorsal stream is responsible for "vision for action" by van der Kamp and colleagues.[41] Successful perception-action or sensorimotor coupling relies on interconnections between the 2 visual streams,[43] and increased functional connectivity between the ventral and dorsal streams is observed during sensorimotor tasks.[44] Importantly, functional connectivity between the visual streams is reduced after a night of sleep deprivation.[39] Furthermore, there are interconnections

between both visual streams and the primary motor cortex, reflecting the importance of the motor cortex in sensorimotor integration and in the sensorimotor coupling process.[45]

Optimal sensorimotor coupling relies on activation of regions that correspond to visual areas (eg, dorsal stream, ventral stream and occipital regions), motor execution, and motor planning/regulation. Increased brain activation in visual and motor regions has been recorded during sensorimotor and perceptual attunement tasks,[40,46,47] and improved sensorimotor coupling in experts may be reflected in their brain activation during such tasks. Bishop and colleagues[46] asked individuals to judge the direction they expected a penalty kick to travel based on videotaped scenes of penalty kicks. Individuals who were more accurate, that is, better able to attune to kinematic cues, had increased activation in areas corresponding to action regulation and perception.[46] Vestibular and proprioceptive inputs regarding whole-body position and joint coordination also contribute to executing an appropriate motor response.[48] For further discussion on the underlying neural processes contributing to sensorimotor function, see the articles by Bishop and colleagues[46] and Yarrow and colleagues.[49]

SLEEP, SLEEP MANIPULATIONS, AND SENSORIMOTOR PERFORMANCE

Sleep extension may contribute to improved sport performance[50] whereas poor sleep (ie, sleep deprivation, restriction, or disruption) and circadian misalignment may compromise performance.[7] Improvements in basketball shooting accuracy[51] and tennis serve accuracy[52] are seen after a sleep extension intervention whereas decrements in basketball shooting accuracy,[53] tennis serve accuracy,[54] and soccer skill[55] are seen after acute sleep restriction and deprivation. To what extent these sleep-related differences in sport performance are due to changes in sensorimotor performance has not been widely studied. Changes in different aspects of sensorimotor performance across laboratory-based tasks, on the other hand, have been investigated under different sleep manipulation protocols: deprivation, restriction, extension, napping, and so forth. Given the multifaceted nature of sensorimotor performance, different tasks target different aspects of sensorimotor performance and provide insight as to how sleep has an impact on these different aspects of sensorimotor performance.

In the sleep field, the psychomotor vigilance task has been widely used to characterize changes in performance capabilities during different sleep manipulation protocols.[8,56] Although the psychomotor vigilance task provides a measure of reaction time and sustained attention and captures elements of sensorimotor function, it does not include an assessment of perceptual judgment and, therefore, may not adequately capture changes in sensorimotor function or behavioral risk relevant to athletes.[8,9,56] Individuals must couple perception of a visual or auditory stimulus with rapid execution of a motor response but the lack of a perceptual judgment or different motor response possibilities limits the functional applicability of the task. Sleep-related changes in other tasks that require perceptual attunement, sensorimotor coupling, or behavioral risk may better capture changes in sensorimotor function.

Performance on saccadic tracking tasks[57] and visual discrimination tasks[58] target oculomotor performance and perceptual attunement, testing whether individuals are able to attune to task-specific features of a visual display. Within such tasks, perceptual performance deteriorates across a period of wakefulness.[57,58] Overnight sleep or daytime naps are needed to restore, and can even enhance, perceptual function.[18,57,59–61] Enhanced perceptual function has been inconsistently observed but may reflect an improved ability to attune to task-specific visual information after sleep.[40] This conclusion is supported by neuroimaging studies finding increased activity in the dorsal stream, ventral stream, and occipital regions during completion of visual discrimination tasks after a night of sleep relative to no intervening sleep.[40,59]

Similar findings have been found across tasks that target motor function, such as finger tapping and tracing tasks. Finger tapping tasks target motor performance and efficient motor control[13] whereas tracing tasks require more sensorimotor coupling.[19] Performance on these sensorimotor tasks is enhanced after sleep, likely reflecting neural plasticity.[13,19] The synaptic remodeling that occurs during sleep, whether through the strengthening of relevant pathways or downscaling of irrelevant pathways, allows for the enhancement of function without additional practice.[13,62] If sleep played only a restorative role, performance would simply return to the prior day's levels and more practice would be needed to improve performance, but that is not the case. During tasks, such as juggling, which have increased temporal constraints, 30-minute naps enhanced performance.[63] Taken together, these findings reflect the importance of sleep to the perception of dynamic features of the environment and to the efficient execution of motor responses.

Sleep deprivation also affects sensorimotor assessments of affordance perception.[25,26] The perception-action coupling task, a novel task developed by Connaboy and colleagues[64] based on the original work of Smith and Pepping,[27] is designed to capture affordance-based behaviors and sensorimotor function and may provide a marker of behavioral risk. Individuals make perceptually based judgements about whether virtual balls can fit through virtual apertures. To perform successfully, they must be attuned to changes in the relative size of the ball and aperture and must accurately perceive what action is afforded based on this relationship. During a study by Connaboy and colleagues,[26] participants were less accurate and responded slower after a night of sleep deprivation. In a separate study using an obstacle negotiation assessment, sleep-deprived individuals underestimated their ability to step over an obstacle while their actual ability to step over the obstacle did not change compared with baseline.[25] These findings are important because the individuals were afforded the same action possibilities when sleep deprived, but they were unable to accurately perceive what actions were afforded to them. Performance on these affordance-based tasks relied on the dynamic updating of perceptual information. Thus, sleep deprivation compromised this aspect of sensorimotor performance.

Sleep may further influence sensorimotor performance by affecting vestibular and somatosensory function, thereby influencing postural control and limb coordination. The link between sleep and vestibular function is reflected by connections between the vestibular system and suprachiasmatic nucleus, an important structure in sleep-wake regulation.[65] The consequences of poor sleep on vestibular function are observed in postural control. Typically, if inaccurate visual information is presented, individuals can decouple their postural responses from this visual input and rely more heavily on vestibular and proprioceptive cues. Under sleep deprivation, individuals are less able to do this suggesting compromised sensorimotor function.[48,66] Because sleep deprivation also alters interjoint coordination, sleep seems to play an important role in ensuring individuals can safely and efficiently execute appropriate motor responses.[15,48,67]

SLEEP FEATURES AND SENSORIMOTOR PERFORMANCE

Understanding that sleep affects performance[7] demonstrates its overall importance but does not explain the mechanism for this effect. Sleep is an active process that varies across the night and between individuals.[68] Improved data recording and analysis techniques, such as high density electroencephalography (EEG) (N ≥64 channels) and quantitative EEG, have allowed more studies to investigate sleep in a granular, feature-specific manner.[68] Different sleep features may relate to different aspects of sensorimotor function. As such, the relationships between specific sleep features/stages and sensorimotor performance need to be addressed.

Sleep Spindles

Sleep spindles are short duration (0.5–3 s) bursts of high-frequency (10–16 Hz) oscillatory activity occurring during non–rapid eye movement (NREM) sleep.[69] Spindles, which arise from the thalamic reticular formation and travel to the cortex through thalamocortical projections,[70] are thought to play an important role in memory consolidation and skill acquisition.[13] Although spindles are distributed across the cortex, increased spindle density is found in frontocentral and centroparietal regions.[68] Corresponding to these increased regions of spindle activity, 2 classes of spindles, slow (approximately 12 Hz) and fast (approximately 14 Hz) have been identified that differ in their spatial distribution on the scalp, temporal distribution throughout the night and functional role.[68,71] Slow spindles are most pronounced in frontal brain regions and occur predominantly during the beginning of the night, often coupling with slow waves in slow wave sleep.[71] Fast spindles are more pronounced in centroparietal regions and occur predominantly toward the end of the night, making up most of the spindles in stage 2 NREM sleep.[71]

Slow spindles have been inconsistently found to contribute to performance on visual discrimination tasks.[18,72] Increased slow spindle-range EEG activity was associated with improved performance on a visual discrimination task after sleep,[18] whereas increased spindle density was associated with worse perceptual learning in a separate study.[72] In contrast, the role of fast spindles has been more consistently defined. Improvements in fine motor tasks, such as finger tapping tasks, were associated with stage 2 sleep in the second half of the night, suggesting a potential role of fast spindles in sensorimotor function.[13,73,74] This role was confirmed in tracing tasks; increased fast spindle density was associated with improved next day performance across different studies in adults[19,75] and children.[17] For example, Tamaki and colleagues[19] found that performance

improvement on the mirror-tracing task was positively associated with fast spindle density, amplitude, and duration but unrelated to slow spindle activity in healthy, young adult participants. Furthermore, during nighttime sleep after practicing novel sensorimotor tasks spindle density,[76] specifically fast spindle density,[75] increased compared to the prepractice night. These findings suggest that fast spindles and the thalamocortical mechanisms responsible for fast spindle generation may be important in sleep-dependent motor skill acquisition and enhancement whereas slow spindles may contribute to perceptual improvements.

Slow Wave Activity

The deepest stage of NREM sleep (N3) is also called slow wave sleep because it is characterized by slow waves. Slow waves are high-amplitude (75 μV), low-frequency (approximately 1 Hz) oscillations that result from cortical neurons alternating between silent states and active states in a coordinated fashion.[69] The silent states and active states correspond to hyperpolarization and depolarization of the cortical neuron cellular membranes, respectively.[70] These waves propagate across the scalp via cortico-cortical connections, typically from frontal regions to more posteriorly located regions.[77] Slow waves are thought to reflect processes contributing to synaptic plasticity and contribute to memory consolidation and learning.[62,78]

Slow wave activity (SWA), NREM EEG power in the 0.5-Hz to 4-Hz range, is also thought to play a role in sensorimotor performance and function. Increased performance on perceptual tasks is associated with increased slow waves from occipital regions[59] whereas performance of sensorimotor tracing tasks has repeatedly resulted in increased SWA in parietal regions during the subsequent night of sleep.[12,16,79] The increase in SWA was specific to brain regions active during task completion and were not observed across the entire scalp.[12] Because parietal brain regions correspond to the dorsal visual stream, SWA enhancement in this region may reflect changes in this stream and may lead to improvements in the ability to act quickly in response to visual information.[12,41] Performance on sensorimotor tasks was improved the next day[12,16,79] and interindividual differences in performance improvement were positively associated with differences in SWA: individuals with more SWA had greater performance improvements.[12] Furthermore, when individuals were deprived of SWA, sensorimotor performance was maintained whereas performance was further enhanced when SWA was increased using auditory stimulation.[16] Conversely, a decrease in sensorimotor function during the day resulted in reduced SWA and reduced motor coordination during the next day.[15] Together, these findings support the notion that SWA plays a critical role in enhancing sensorimotor performance through influencing sensory and motor aspects of performance.

Rapid Eye Movement Sleep

Rapid eye movement (REM) sleep consists of low-amplitude, mixed-frequency waves that resemble wake and likely plays a role in memory consolidation.[69] Disruption of REM sleep has an impact on the excitability of hippocampal neurons, impairing long-term potentiation and subsequent memory formation.[78] Relevant to sensorimotor function, muscle twitches are common during REM sleep in infants and children.[80,81] These muscle twitches are associated with brain activity in regions related to sensorimotor function, such as the hippocampus, cerebellum, and red nucleus.[80] As such, REM sleep may be important to the development of the sensorimotor system and to the integration between the sensory and motor systems. REM muscle twitches are found into adulthood although their function in adulthood has not been investigated.[81] Beyond likely playing a role in the development of an integrated sensorimotor system, REM sleep also influences daily changes in sensorimotor performance. Interindividual differences in REM sleep contributed to different levels of improvement in a visual discrimination task.[59] Increased REM sleep resulted in greater performance improvements.[59]

FUTURE DIRECTIONS

Although much has been learned about the relationship between sleep and sensorimotor performance, there are several areas that need to be further addressed. Affordance-based tasks have been widely studied in different sport-specific scenarios, but perception-action coupling and sensorimotor performance are important aspects of function across different professions. Sensorimotor performance is essential for truck drivers merging into traffic, surgeons performing operations, and military personnel executing missions, all of whom may be operating while sleep restricted. Studying profession-relevant aspects of sensorimotor performance within these populations would provide valuable insight into how their performance may be optimized or how sleep interventions may be developed to help minimize sleep loss.

Furthermore, different sleep features have been associated with sensorimotor performance enhancement. Unfortunately, the tasks used in many of these studies have been laboratory-based tasks and have not been representative of real-world scenarios. Further work is needed to confirm the functional relevance of different sleep features on sport-specific sensorimotor function using representative sensorimotor assessments. As more sleep features associated with sensorimotor performance are identified, the natural question that follows is whether these features can be induced to facilitate performance improvements. Because SWA and sleep spindles have been implicated as an important indicator of performance improvements across different cognitive domains, increasing those sleep features has been the subject of different sleep optimization interventions.[82,83] The timely administration of tones through a closed loop system has proved to increase SWA[83,84] as well as sleep spindles,[82] but it is not known whether this enhancement in sleep-specific EEG oscillations may ameliorate function in the same way as those occurring naturally.

SUMMARY

The sensorimotor system involves a tight functional coupling between sensory and motor functions, which is essential for sports performance. Describing sensorimotor performance from an ecological dynamics perspective provides an understanding of the dynamic and continuous nature of this coupling defined within the interaction between the individual and environment. Sleep may play a role across different aspects of sensorimotor function, having an impact on sensory function, motor function, and sensorimotor coupling. Furthermore, specific features of sleep, namely spindles and slow waves, seem to play a critical role in sensorimotor function. Understanding how these sleep features influence sport-specific tasks may provide greater insight into how sleep affects sensorimotor coupling and sport performance.

DISCLOSURE

The authors have nothing to disclose.

REFERENCES

1. Knufinke M, Nieuwenhuys A, Geurts SAE, et al. Self-reported sleep quantity, quality and sleep hygiene in elite athletes. J Sleep Res 2018;27(1):78–85.
2. Roberts SSH, Teo WP, Warmington SA. Effects of training and competition on the sleep of elite athletes: a systematic review and meta-analysis. Br J Sports Med 2019;53(8):513–22.

3. Fowler PM, Knez W, Crowcroft S, et al. Greater effect of East versus west travel on jet lag, sleep, and team sport performance. Med Sci Sports Exerc 2017; 49(12):2548–61.

4. Lastella M, Roach GD, Sargent C. Travel fatigue and sleep/wake behaviors of professional soccer players during international competition. Sleep Health 2019; 5(2):141–7.

5. Sargent C, Halson S, Roach GD. Sleep or swim? Early-morning training severely restricts the amount of sleep obtained by elite swimmers. Eur J Sport Sci 2014;14(Suppl 1):S310–5.

6. Shearer DA, Jones RM, Kilduff LP, et al. Effects of competition on the sleep patterns of elite rugby union players. Eur J Sport Sci 2015;15(8):681–6.

7. Fullagar HH, Skorski S, Duffield R, et al. Sleep and athletic performance: the effects of sleep loss on exercise performance, and physiological and cognitive responses to exercise. Sports Med 2015;45(2): 161–86.

8. Lim J, Dinges DF. A meta-analysis of the impact of short-term sleep deprivation on cognitive variables. Psychol Bull 2010;136(3):375–89.

9. Harpham JA, Mihalik JP, Littleton AC, et al. The effect of visual and sensory performance on head impact biomechanics in college football players. Ann Biomed Eng 2014;42(1):1–10.

10. Burris K, Vittetoe K, Ramger B, et al. Sensorimotor abilities predict on-field performance in professional baseball. Sci Rep 2018;8(1):116.

11. Poltavski D, Biberdorf D. The role of visual perception measures used in sports vision programmes in predicting actual game performance in Division I collegiate hockey players. J Sports Sci 2015;33(6): 597–608.

12. Huber R, Ghilardi MF, Massimini M, et al. Local sleep and learning. Nature 2004;430(6995): 78–81.

13. Walker MP, Brakefield T, Morgan A, et al. Practice with sleep makes perfect: sleep-dependent motor skill learning. Neuron 2002;35(1):205–11.

14. Walker MP, Stickgold R. It's practice, with sleep, that makes perfect: implications of sleep-dependent learning and plasticity for skill performance. Clin Sports Med 2005;24(2):301–17, ix.

15. Huber R, Ghilardi MF, Massimini M, et al. Arm immobilization causes cortical plastic changes and locally decreases sleep slow wave activity. Nat Neurosci 2006;9(9):1169–76.

16. Landsness EC, Crupi D, Hulse BK, et al. Sleep-dependent improvement in visuomotor learning: a causal role for slow waves. Sleep 2009;32(10): 1273–84.

17. Astill RG, Piantoni G, Raymann RJ, et al. Sleep spindle and slow wave frequency reflect motor skill performance in primary school-age children. Front Hum Neurosci 2014;8:910.

18. Bang JW, Khalilzadeh O, Hamalainen M, et al. Location specific sleep spindle activity in the early visual areas and perceptual learning. Vision Res 2014;99: 162–71.

19. Tamaki M, Matsuoka T, Nittono H, et al. Fast sleep spindle (13-15 hz) activity correlates with sleep-dependent improvement in visuomotor performance. Sleep 2008;31(2):204–11.

20. Gibson J. The ecological approach to visual perception. Boston: Houghton Mifflin; 1979.

21. Fajen BR, Matthis JS. Direct perception of action-scaled affordances: the shrinking gap problem. J Exp Psychol Hum Percept Perform 2011;37(5): 1442–57.

22. Davids K, Button C, Araujo D, et al. Movement models from sports provide representative task constrains for studying adaptive behavior in human movement systems. Adapt Behav 2006;14(1):73–95.

23. Fajen BR, Riley MA, Turvey MT. Information, affordances, and the control of action in sport. Int J Sport Psychol 2008;40:79–107.

24. Sarpeshkar V, Mann DL. Biomechanics and visual-motor control: how it has, is, and will be used to reveal the secrets of hitting a cricket ball. Sports Biomech 2011;10(4):306–23.

25. Daviaux Y, Mignardot JB, Cornu C, et al. Effects of total sleep deprivation on the perception of action capabilities. Exp Brain Res 2014;232(7):2243–53.

26. Connaboy C, LaGoy AD, Johnson CD, et al. Sleep deprivation impairs affordance perception behavior during an action boundary accuracy assessment. Acta Astronaut 2020;166:270–6.

27. Smith J, Pepping GJ. Effects of affordance perception on the initiation and actualization of action. Ecol Psychol 2010;22:119–49.

28. Eagle SR, Kontos AP, Pepping GJ, et al. Increased risk of musculoskeletal injury following sport-related concussion: a perception-action coupling approach. Sports Med 2019. [Epub ahead of print].

29. Eagle SR, Nindl BC, Johnson CD, et al. Does concussion affect perception-action coupling behavior? Action boundary perception as a biomarker for concussion. Clin J Sport Med 2019. [Epub ahead of print].

30. Cordovil R, Araújo D, Pepping G-J, et al. An ecological stance on risk and safe behaviors in children: the role of affordances and emergent behaviors. New Ideas Psychol 2015;36:50–9.

31. Dicks M, Button C, Davids K. Examination of gaze behaviors under in situ and video simulation task constraints reveals differences in information pickup for perception and action. Atten Percept Psychophys 2010;72(3):706–20.

32. Farrow D, Abernethy B. Do expertise and the degree of perception-action coupling affect natural anticipatory performance? Perception 2003; 32(9):1127–39.

33. Stone JA, Maynard IW, North JS, et al. Emergent perception-action couplings regulate postural adjustments during performance of externally-timed dynamic interceptive actions. Psychol Res 2015; 79(5):829–43.

34. Mann DL, Spratford W, Abernethy B. The head tracks and gaze predicts: how the world's best batters hit a ball. PLoS One 2013;8(3):e58289.

35. Ranganathan R, Carlton LG. Perception-action coupling and anticipatory performance in baseball batting. J Mot Behav 2007;39(5):369–80.

36. Panchuk D, Davids K, Sakadjian A, et al. Did you see that? Dissociating advanced visual information and ball flight constrains perception and action processes during one-handed catching. Acta Psychol (Amst) 2013;142(3):394–401.

37. Bootsma RJ, van Wieringen PCW. Timing an attacking forehand drive in table tennis. J Exp Psychol Hum Percept Perform 1990;16(1):21–9.

38. Tong J, Maruta J, Heaton KJ, et al. Adaptation of visual tracking synchronization after one night of sleep deprivation. Exp Brain Res 2014;232(1): 121–31.

39. Lim J, Tan JC, Parimal S, et al. Sleep deprivation impairs object-selective attention: a view from the ventral visual cortex. PLoS One 2010;5(2):e9087.

40. Walker MP, Stickgold R, Jolesz FA, et al. The functional anatomy of sleep-dependent visual skill learning. Cereb Cortex 2005;15(11):1666–75.

41. van der Kamp J, Rivas F, Doorn H, et al. Ventral and dorsal system contributions to visual anticipation in fast ball sports. Int J Sport Psychol 2008;39:100–30.

42. Lamme VA, Roelfsema PR. The distinct modes of vision offered by feedforward and recurrent processing. Trends Neurosci 2000;23(11):571–9.

43. Milner AD. How do the two visual streams interact with each other? Exp Brain Res 2017;235(5): 1297–308.

44. Hutchison RM, Gallivan JP. Functional coupling between frontoparietal and occipitotemporal pathways during action and perception. Cortex 2018;98:8–27.

45. Calderon CB, Van Opstal F, Peigneux P, et al. Task-relevant information modulates primary motor cortex activity before movement onset. Front Hum Neurosci 2018;12:93.

46. Bishop DT, Wright MJ, Jackson RC, et al. Neural bases for anticipation skill in soccer: an FMRI study. J Sport Exerc Psychol 2013;35(1):98–109.

47. Maquet P, Schwartz S, Passingham R, et al. Sleep-related consolidation of a visuomotor skill: brain mechanisms as assessed by functional magnetic resonance imaging. J Neurosci 2003;23(4):1432–40.

48. Aguiar SA, Barela JA. Adaptation of sensorimotor coupling in postural control is impaired by sleep deprivation. PLoS One 2015;10(3):e0122340.

49. Yarrow K, Brown P, Krakauer JW. Inside the brain of an elite athlete: the neural processes that support

high achievement in sports. Nat Rev Neurosci 2009;10(8):585–96.

50. Bonnar D, Bartel K, Kakoschke N, et al. Sleep interventions designed to improve athletic performance and recovery: a systematic review of current approaches. Sports Med 2018;48(3): 683–703.

51. Mah CD, Mah KE, Kezirian EJ, et al. The effects of sleep extension on the athletic performance of collegiate basketball players. Sleep 2011;34(7):943–50.

52. Schwartz J, Simon RD Jr. Sleep extension improves serving accuracy: a study with college varsity tennis players. Physiol Behav 2015;151:541–4.

53. Jones JJ, Kirschen GW, Kancharla S, et al. Association between late-night tweeting and next-day game performance among professional basketball players. Sleep Health 2019;5(1):68–71.

54. Reyner LA, Horne JA. Sleep restriction and serving accuracy in performance tennis players, and effects of caffeine. Physiol Behav 2013;120:93–6.

55. Pallesen S, Gundersen HS, Kristoffersen M, et al. The effects of sleep deprivation on soccer skills. Percept Mot Skills 2017;124(4):812–29.

56. Drummond SP, Bischoff-Grethe A, Dinges DF, et al. The neural basis of the psychomotor vigilance task. Sleep 2005;28(9):1059–68.

57. Gais S, Koster S, Sprenger A, et al. Sleep is required for improving reaction times after training on a procedural visuo-motor task. Neurobiol Learn Mem 2008;90(4):610–5.

58. Mednick SC, Arman AC, Boynton GM. The time course and specificity of perceptual deterioration. Proc Natl Acad Sci U S A 2005;102(10):3881–5.

59. Mascetti L, Muto V, Matarazzo L, et al. The impact of visual perceptual learning on sleep and local slow-wave initiation. J Neurosci 2013;33(8):3323–31.

60. Mednick SC, Drummond SP, Arman AC, et al. Perceptual deterioration is reflected in the neural response: fMRI study of nappers and non-nappers. Perception 2008;37(7):1086–97.

61. Mednick SC, Nakayama K, Cantero JL, et al. The restorative effect of naps on perceptual deterioration. Nat Neurosci 2002;5(7):677–81.

62. Tononi G, Cirelli C. Sleep and the price of plasticity: from synaptic and cellular homeostasis to memory consolidation and integration. Neuron 2014;81(1): 12–34.

63. Morita Y, Ogawa K, Uchida S. Napping after complex motor learning enhances juggling performance. Sleep Sci 2016;9(2):112–6.

64. Connaboy C, Johnson CD, LaGoy AD, et al. Inter-session reliability and within-session stability of a novel perception-action coupling task. Aerosp Med Hum Perform 2019;90(2):77–83.

65. Besnard S, Tighilet B, Chabbert C, et al. The balance of sleep: role of the vestibular sensory system. Sleep Med Rev 2018;42:220–8.

66. Cheng S, Ma J, Sun J, et al. Differences in sensory reweighting due to loss of visual and proprioceptive cues in postural stability support among sleep-deprived cadet pilots. Gait Posture 2018;63:97–103.

67. Mah CD, Sparks AJ, Samaan MA, et al. Sleep restriction impairs maximal jump performance and joint coordination in elite athletes. J Sports Sci 2019;1–8.

68. Cox R, Schapiro AC, Manoach DS, et al. Individual differences in frequency and topography of slow and fast sleep spindles. Front Hum Neurosci 2017;11:433.

69. Iber C, American Academy of Sleep Medicine. The AASM manual for the scoring of sleep and associated events: rules, terminology and technical specifications. Westchester (IL): American Academy of Sleep Medicine; 2007.

70. Steriade M. The corticothalamic system in sleep. Front Biosci 2003;8:d878–99.

71. Jobert M, Poiseau E, Jahnig P, et al. Topographical analysis of sleep spindle activity. Neuropsychobiology 1992;26(4):210–7.

72. Mednick SC, McDevitt EA, Walsh JK, et al. The critical role of sleep spindles in hippocampal-dependent memory: a pharmacology study. J Neurosci 2013;33(10):4494–504.

73. Plihal W, Born J. Effects of early and late nocturnal sleep on declarative and procedural memory. J Cogn Neurosci 1997;9(4):534–47.

74. Piantoni G, Halgren E, Cash SS. The contribution of thalamocortical core and matrix pathways to sleep spindles. Neural Plast 2016;2016:3024342.

75. Tamaki M, Matsuoka T, Nittono H, et al. Activation of fast sleep spindles at the premotor cortex and parietal areas contributes to motor learning: a study using sLORETA. Clin Neurophysiol 2009;120(5):878–86.

76. Fogel SM, Smith CT. Learning-dependent changes in sleep spindles and Stage 2 sleep. J Sleep Res 2006;15(3):250–5.

77. Massimini M, Huber R, Ferrarelli F, et al. The sleep slow oscillation as a traveling wave. J Neurosci 2004;24(31):6862–70.

78. Walker MP, Stickgold R. Sleep, memory, and plasticity. Annu Rev Psychol 2006;57:139–66.

79. Landsness EC, Ferrarelli F, Sarasso S, et al. Electrophysiological traces of visuomotor learning and their renormalization after sleep. Clin Neurophysiol 2011;122(12):2418–25.

80. Peever J, Fuller PM. The biology of REM sleep. Curr Biol 2017;27(22):R1237–48.

81. Blumberg MS. Developing sensorimotor systems in our sleep. Curr Dir Psychol Sci 2015;24(1):32–7.

82. Antony JW, Paller KA. Using oscillating sounds to manipulate sleep spindles. Sleep 2017;40(3).

83. Wilckens KA, Ferrarelli F, Walker MP, et al. Slow-wave activity enhancement to improve cognition. Trends Neurosci 2018;41(7):470–82.

84. Garcia-Molina G, Tsoneva T, Jasko J, et al. Closed-loop system to enhance slow-wave activity. J Neural Eng 2018;15(6):066018.

Sleep and Athletic Performance
Impacts on Physical Performance, Mental Performance, Injury Risk and Recovery, and Mental Health

Jonathan Charest[a,b], Michael A. Grandner, PhD, MTR[c,*]

KEYWORDS

• Sleep • Sport • Insomnia • Performance

KEY POINTS

• Insufficient sleep and poor sleep quality are prevalent among athletes, potentially due to time demands, physical demands, and developmental needs.
• Sleep disturbances among athletes have adverse impacts on physical performance, mental performance, injury risk and recovery, medical health, and mental health.
• Sleep interventions among athletes have been shown to improve physical strength and speed, cognitive performance and reaction time, mental health, and other domains.
• Sport organizations should incorporate sleep health promotion programs at individual, team, and system levels.

INTRODUCTION
Scope of the Problem

In recent years, there has been increased attention toward the importance of sleep and its essential role in athletic performance, cognition, health, and mental well-being. Many of these studies examine elite athletes (eg, Olympians, professionals, and/or players recruited to national and varsity teams) and some focus on athletes in general. Despite all the efforts expended, by any definition, numerous athletes still experience inadequate sleep.[1–3] Compared with nonathletes, athletes tend to sleep less on average.[4] Furthermore, athletes' quality of sleep seems lower than their nonathlete peers.[5–7] Additionally, it has been suggested that certain types of athletes are more prone to developing sleep difficulties, such

as sleep apnea. For example, according to George and colleagues[8] and Albuquerque and colleagues,[9] National Football League (NFL) players have higher rates of obstructive sleep apnea, which have tremendous deleterious impacts on health and daytime sleepiness. There is increasing evidence that poor sleep is a good predictor for injuries and, more importantly, concussion.[10]

Position Statements

Recently, the International Olympic Committee (IOC), has addressed, for the first time, sleep as a major contributor to athletic performance and as a fundamental feature of athlete mental health.[11,12] In addition, the National Collegiate Athletics Association (NCAA)[13–17] included sleep health as part of their published mental health

---

[a] Department of Psychology, Universite Laval, Quebec City, Quebec, Canada; [b] Centre for Sleep and Human Performance, #106, 51 Sunpark Drive Southeast, Calgary, Alberta T2X 3V4, Canada; [c] Department of Psychiatry, University of Arizona, 1501 North Campbell Avenue, PO Box 245002, Tucson, AZ 8524-5002, USA
* Corresponding author.
E-mail address: grandner@gmail.com

Sleep Med Clin 15 (2020) 41–57
https://doi.org/10.1016/j.jsmc.2019.11.005

best practices[18] as well as their more recently published official position statement on the importance of sleep health for student athletes.[18] These position statements from the NCAA and IOC represent the increased awareness of the importance of sleep health among organizations of elite athletes. Both of these documents were the result of a literature review, Delphi process of iterative consensus building, and subsequent revision, after exhaustive reviews of available literature.

The IOC mental health document[11] considers sleep health in terms of sufficiency (ie, at least 7 hours for adults), proper circadian alignment, good overall perceived sleep quality, and absence of sleep disorders, including insomnia disorder and sleep apnea. The document recommends that these dimensions of sleep be considered important for mental health as well as physical health and functioning. Furthermore, the document recommends education, proper assessment and screening, and treatment using evidence-based strategies—given the consideration that some treatments may have an impact on safety and/or performance.

The NCAA document focused on sleep as an important aspect of health, performance, and mental functioning in collegiate student athletes.[18] It addresses many identified barriers to sleep, including academic, athletic, and social time demands. Similarly, this document defines sleep health in terms of duration (at least 7 hours in adults), timing, overall quality, and absence of disorders, including insomnia and sleep apnea. Particular attention also is paid to the role of tiredness, fatigue, and/or sleepiness as consequences of sleep loss and/or disturbances. The NCAA makes 5 recommendations in this document:

1. Conduct a collegiate athlete time demands survey annually.
2. Ensure that consumer sleep technology, if used, is compliant with Health Insurance Portability and Accountability Act and Family Educational Rights and Privacy Act laws.
3. Incorporate sleep screening into the preparticipation examination.
4. Provide collegiate athletes with evidence-based sleep education that includes (1) information on sleep best practices, (2) information about the role of sleep in optimizing athletic and academic performance and overall well-being, and (3) strategies for addressing sleep barriers.
5. Provide coaches with evidence-based sleep education that includes (1) information on sleep best practices, (2) information about the role of sleep in optimizing athletic and academic performance and overall well-being, and (3) strategies to help optimize collegiate athlete sleep.

These efforts specifically recommend that sleep-related education should be provided, sleep difficulties and disorders should be routinely assessed and screened for, and sleep health promotion should be a goal of athletics programs.

EPIDEMIOLOGY OF SLEEP DISTURBANCES IN ATHLETES
Prevalence of Insufficient Sleep

Insufficient sleep duration can have an impact on metabolism, endocrine function, and athletic and cognitive outcomes, and, furthermore, increase perceived effort during exercise.[19–21] When athletes are compared with nonathletes, they tend to sleep less and less efficiently. Leeder and colleagues[4] compared the habits of 47 elite athletes over a 4-day period to a group of nonathletes, using actigraphy; ages of participants were not reported, but groups were matched for age and gender. On average, athletes slept 6.55 hours $\pm$ 0.43 hours versus 7.11 hours $\pm$ 0.25 hours in the nonathletes ($P = .27$). They did report, however, lower sleep efficiency (80.6 hours $\pm$ 6.4 hours vs 88.7 hours $\pm$ 3.6 hours; $P<.05$), higher time spent in bed (8:07 hours $\pm$ 0:20 hours vs 8:36 hours $\pm$ 0.53 hours; $P<.05$), wake after sleep onset (0:50 hours $\pm$ 0:16 hours vs 1:17 hours $\pm$ 0:31 hours; $P<.05$), sleep-onset latency (5.0 hours $\pm$ 2.5 hours vs 18.2 hours $\pm$ 16.5 hours; $P<.05$), and sleep fragmentation (29.8 hours $\pm$ 9.0 hours vs 36.0 hours $\pm$ 12.4 hours; $P<.05$) in athletes. Furthermore, Lastella and colleagues[22] reported insufficient sleep duration among athletes, with 6.8 hours on average. Sargent and colleagues[23,24] also reported that over 14 nights assessed with actigraphy, athletes recorded an average of 6.5 hours of sleep per night.

Taken together, these studies have investigated a total of 241 elite athletes and, documented actigraphically, determined sleep durations of approximately 6.5 hours in most cases. Recently, Mah and colleagues[25] indicated that 39.1% of athletes reported insufficient sleep (<7 hours) by self-report. And, among a large sample of collegiate athletes in the United States (N = 8312), Turner and colleagues[26] reported that the mean number of nights per week that athletes did not think they got enough sleep was 3.8.

Prevalence of Poor Sleep Quality

Hoshikawa and colleagues[27] investigated the quality of sleep of 817 Japanese elite athletes with the Pittsburgh Sleep Quality Index (PSQI), showing that 28% of the participants exhibited a score greater than 5, suggesting poor quality of sleep. Mah and colleagues[25] reported that 42.2% of the 629 athletes in that study experienced poor sleep quality, also using the PSQI. In 2019, Turner and colleagues[26] examined data from 8312 collegiate student athletes and found that 19.8% reported that "sleep difficulties" were particularly "traumatic or difficult to handle" over the past 12 months and that 21.8% reported extreme difficulty falling asleep at least 3 nights per week. Bleyer and colleagues[5] reported that 38% of their 452 participants reported poor sleep. Findings from a study conducted among elite rugby and cricket players (n = 175) showed that 50% of their participants' PSQI score were greater than 5 and that 9% scored greater than 10.[3] Tsunoda and colleagues[7] reported the PSQI scores of 14 wheelchair basketball athletes (mean = 5.8 ± 3.0) and compared their results with 103 nonathletes from the general population (mean = 4.51 ± 2.14). Regardless of total sleep time, the wheelchair athletes reported lower sleep quality and lower sleep efficiency than matched nonathletes.

In a cohort of 317 athletes from the Rio de Janeiro 2016 Summer Olympics from 11 different sports, poor sleep quality (as assessed by the PSQI) was prevalent in more than 50% of the athletes after the Olympic Games.[28] This research recapitulates the earlier results with a similar cohort, in which up to 83% of athletes reach the cutoff, indicating poor sleep.[29] The higher proportion with a score greater than 5 occurred in the lead-up to the Olympics and the lower figure was recorded at the games. Consequently, regardless of the type of sports, these results highlight the prevalence of poor sleep quality among athletes.

Prevalence of Daytime Sleepiness

Few studies have examined the prevalence of general fatigue and/or sleepiness among athletes. Turner and colleagues[26] reported that 60.9% of collegiate athletes report that they experience feeling "tired, dragged out, or sleepy during the day" at least 3 days per week (as measured by self-report). Furthermore, 32.75% of these collegiate student athletes reported an inability to maintain wakefulness at least 3 times per week (by self-report). Mah and colleagues[25] reported that 51% of student athletes in their study reported high scores (≥10) on the Epworth Sleepiness Scale. These findings indicate high levels of sleepiness in elite athletes.

Prevalence of Circadian Preferences and Disruption

Data exploring chronotype among the general population suggest that approximately 25% are morning types, 50% are intermediate types, and approximately 25% are evening types.[30] Few studies have explored the chronotype distribution among athletes. Two studies[2,31] indicated that 51% of athletes were classified as morning types, 40% as intermediate types, and only 9% were classified as evening types. One study examined athletes in wheelchairs and the other examined school-aged athletes and may not be representative of the elite athlete population. Lastella and colleagues[32] investigated 114 elite athletes emerging from 5 different sports. Their results indicated that 28% were morning types, 65% were intermediate types, and only 6% were evening types, supporting previous findings that athletes tend to pursue and excel in sports that match their chronotype.[33]

Circadian rhythms can influence variations in performance, depending on the time of day and typical training schedules, which ultimately can affect competitive performance.[34] When athletes experience disturbances in their environments or routines, such as overnight travel, repetitive time zone changes, evening training, or late-night competition, endogenous circadian rhythms and normal sleep patterns may be out of synchrony.[35,36] Such disruptions in circadian and sleep patterns can increase homeostatic pressure and thus influence the regulation of emotions, body temperature, and circulation of melatonin and cause a significant increase in sleep latency.[37] The sleep/wake behavior of athletes often is governed by their training schedules.[38] Therefore, the role of chronotype among athletes may interact with a training schedule and should be considered to optimize training and performance[34] and reduce the prevalence of chronobiologic disturbances.

Prevalence of Sleep Disorders

Insomnia

Gupta and colleagues[39] demonstrated that the relation between elite sport participation and insomnia symptomology is poorly systematized. Daytime impairment—a key part of insomnia diagnosis—can reflect a wide variety of experiences, including fatigue, emotional fluctuation, and psychomotor and/or neuropsychological performance, which all are important for elite athletes. Given this particular sensitivity to performance impairment and high levels of sleepiness (which is not common in insomnia), there arise some challenges in insomnia assessment among elite athletes. Traditional insomnia models might poorly discriminate insomnia per se in this nontraditional population.[40] The multifaceted demands of elite sport, including a high level of training volume,[41,42] precompetition anxiety,[22,38,43] and circadian challenges (jet lag)[44] all can predispose and precipitate sleep disturbance, thus leading to or facilitating symptomology of insomnia.

Given the absence of a validated sleep questionnaire specifically for athletes before the creation of the Athlete Sleep Screening Questionnaire (ASSQ),[45] it is difficult to precisely indicate the insomnia prevalence in elite athletes. The systematic review conducted by Gupta and colleagues,[39] however, reported that sleep disturbance complaints range from 13% to 70% of the athletes and that overall, on average, 26% of the athletes significantly scored for insomnia symptoms using the Insomnia Severity Index and PSQI. It Notwithstanding the popularity of these 2 questionnaires, neither of them is specifically validated in an elite athlete population. Elite athletes are selected primarily not only on the basis of physiologic predisposition but also psychological attributes.[46,47] It is possible that personality traits that include a focus on success (eg, perfectionism) also may predispose an elite athlete to insomnia.[48] Furthermore, the demands of elite sports, including an elevated frequency, intensity, and volume of activity and scheduling challenges,[23,42] coupled with precompetition anxiety[43] and jetlag/travel,[49,50] may all lead an individual toward sleep difficulties. Given that these challenges are uncommon among the general population and the relationship between risk factors and sleep may be fundamentally different in this group (eg, distribution of muscle mass), tools not specifically validated in athletic populations should be used somewhat cautiously.

Sleep apnea

The prevalence of sleep apnea may be high in certain type of sports, such as strength, power, and high-contact sports, where athletes often present with a large body mass and neck circumference.[3,51,52] In the NFL and National Hockey League, 2 high-speed and high-contact sports, an elevated body mass index and a large neck circumference are considered protective assets, making athletes less injury-prone.[3] These specific body traits, however, unfortunately, also predispose these athletes to an increased risk of obstructive sleep apnea (OSA).[52–54] Two studies carried out among NFL players illustrated that players with these specific physical traits seemed to have a higher incidence of OSA.[8,55] Additionally, in line with the previous football studies, Dobrosielski and colleagues[56] illustrated that

approximately 8% of the NCAA Division I football players were at risk for OSA. Moreover, in professional hockey players, OSA was present in approximately 10% of athletes.[57] It is reported that, in most cases, the OSA severity was mild but even mild OSA might cause major disturbances in sleep,[58] potentially having an impact athletic performance.

Other disorders

Few studies have been conducted on restless legs syndrome (RLS) among athletes. Findings from a study assessing a population of runners indicate prevalence is suggested at approximately 13%.[59] Among hockey players, prevalence is suggested at approximately 5%[57]; finally, within a sample of rugby players, no participants reported RLS but 12% reported periodic limb movements (PLMs).[60] These 2 studies have shown that sleep disorders, such as RLS and PLMs, are relatively common among elite athletes from a variety of sports.

IMPACT OF SLEEP ON PHYSICAL PERFORMANCE

Adverse effects of sleep restriction on athletic performance have been documented for many years, including cardiorespiratory and psychomotor effects, which require sustained and stable performance over time.[61–65] Mougin[65] observed 7 participants on a cycle ergometer, in a study that included a 10-minute warm-up and then a 20-minute steady exercise corresponding to 75% of the predetermined maximal oxygen consumption and was followed by an increased-intensity exercise until exhaustion. This was done along with sleep restriction (3 hours of wakefulness in the middle of the night). In this study, physiologic demands were significantly higher during the submaximal effort compared with a baseline night (10:30 PM to 7:00 AM).[65] Heart rate was significantly higher when measured after 9 minutes (167.1 bpm ± 2.0 vs 171.3 bpm ± 2.5) and after 20 minutes (176.0 bpm ± 2.6 vs 179.1 bpm± 2.4). Also, ventilation (141.0 bpm ± 5.7 vs 157.5 bpm ± 6.4) and respiratory frequency (43.0 bpm ± 1.6 vs 44.7 bpm ± 1.7) were both altered after a sleep restriction compared with baseline. Similarly, these same variables were significantly higher after the sleep restriction condition when performing a graded exercise stress test, until exhaustion, whereas the volume of maximal oxygen uptake ($V_{O_{2max}}$) decreased. Lactate accumulation was also greater at the ninth minute ($P<.01$), at the twentieth minute ($P<.05$) of the steady power exercise, and at maximal exercise

(P<.05) after sleep restriction. These results from Mougin[65] elegantly demonstrated that after a sleep restriction, physical performances require a higher physiologic demand, ultimately leading the athletes to exhaustion faster than he should have been. In a separate study, however, there was no significant change in mean or maximal power in anaerobic tests after a 3:00 AM bedtime compared with a 10:30 PM bedtime.[66] Subsequent studies by Mougin showed that after 4-hours' sleep restriction, the maximum work rate developed by the participants was reduced by 15 W for cyclists in a 30-minute exercise at 75% of maximum power.[67] In agreement with some of the previous results, the average and maximum powers of an anaerobic test decrease among students,[68] football players,[69] and judokas[70] after a single 4-hour sleep restriction. The reasoning behind the decrease in resistance to exercise is the alteration of the aerobic pathways[64] or in the perceptual change (impression of a longer effort), because the physiologic aspects remain predominantly unchanged.[62,63] The increase in perceived effort accompanied by a reduction in generated power supports the theory of neuromuscular fatigue,[71] possibly indicating a combination of central nervous system response and neural theory of sleep.[62,72,73]

Other studies also have shown adverse impacts of sleep restriction on athletes' anaerobic power,[74] tennis serving accuracy,[75] isometric force,[76] and cortisol levels.[77] In addition, the average distance traveled by elite runners decreases (6.224–6.037 miles) in a treadmill exercise (30 minutes) at their own pace.[78] Skein and colleagues[79] reported lower average sprint times, reduced glycogen concentration in the muscles, and decreased strength and activation during an isometric force test after a 30-hour total sleep deprivation, with 10 athletes from team sports, compared with a normal 8 hours of sleep. Submaximal-effort sports, such as running, might be more likely affected by total sleep deprivation than maximum-effort sports, such as weightlifting, because they require more time and, therefore, have a negative impact on the perception of effort throughout time perhaps due to the higher physiologic demand required.[65] After sleep restriction, the perception of effort increases exponentially increased completion time of the test.[78] The differences in muscle contraction results (voluntary activation), however, can probably be explained by the sensitivity and accuracy of the electromyography equipment used. For example, previous studies probably have been limited in this aspect contrary to recent studies due to the technological advancement of equipment.[79,80] In summary, although the effects of sleep deprivation on exercise are not completely understood, many converging results imply adverse effects of sleep deprivation on athletic performance.

Moreover, the balance of the energy substrate seems vulnerable to sleep deprivation. For instance, a 30-hour sleep deprivation compared with an 8-hour sleep opportunity demonstrated the inability of the human body to fully recover (24 hours) muscle glycogen in an athletic population, as shown by the muscle glycogen concentration before exercise (310 mmol*kg^{-1} dw $\pm$ 67 mmol*kg^{-1} dw vs 209 mmol*kg^{-1} dw $\pm$ 60 mmol*kg^{-1} dw).[79] Inadequate glucose intake would hinder athletes' ability to compete for extended periods, because glycogen shortage is known to reduce muscle function and athletic stamina.[81,82] It seems that a large energy imbalance leads to a deterioration in both aerobic and anaerobic power production when activity is sustained over several days and sleep is reduced.[83–87] Prolonged periods of sleep deprivation are associated with increased sympathetic nervous system activity and decreases in parasympathetic nervous system activity as well as altered spontaneous baroreflex sensitivity during vigilance testing in healthy adults.[88] Because disturbances of sympathetic and parasympathetic equilibrium are associated with overtraining,[89] it is possible that these disturbances of the autonomic nervous system after sleep deprivation may promote the development of a state of overtraining in athletes.[82,90] Despite these nervous system disturbances, several studies have reported that sleep deprivation has minimal impact on the cardiorespiratory variables during exercise,[62,66,91] as opposed to the previous finding of Mougin and colleagues.[65] Differences probably are more attributable to the protocols administered and the exercise mode used (running, cycling, and time of exhaustion) throughout these different studies. In addition to these results, there were no significant effects on cardiorespiratory or thermoregulatory function in athletes despite a reduction in the distance run for 30 minutes on a treadmill after sleep deprivation.[78] Oliver[78] hypothesized the minimal effects on cardiorespiratory function could be due to the influence of perceived effort during the final stages of prolonged high-intensity exercise (described previously).

IMPACT OF SLEEP ON INJURY RISK AND RECOVERY
Sleep and Concussions

It is estimated that as many as 3.8 million concussions are sustained in the United States during competitive sports per year.[92] Regrettably, approximately 50% of concussions may go unreported.[92] As many as 1 million student athletes reported having 2 or more concussions during a period of 12 months.[93] A study indicated that 40% of athletes with a concussion reported that their coaches were not aware of their symptoms.[94] Moreover, it is suggested that athletes involved in team sports have significantly higher risk for 1 or more concussions than athletes in individual sports.[93]

Sleep may play an important role as a risk factor for concussions. Participants were given sleep screening questionnaires and followed over a 1-year period. Predictors of incident concussions included clinically moderate to severe insomnia (relative risk [RR] 3.13; 95% CI, 1.320–7.424; $P = .015$) and excessive daytime sleepiness (RR 2.856; 95% CI, 0.681–11.977; $P = .037$), in a study of 190 NCAA athletes,[10] and these risk factors outperformed more traditional risk factors (eg, high-risk sport and history of concussions) as predictors.

Postconcussion sleep also is important. Recently, a meta-analysis reported that sleep disturbances were reported after a concussion approximately 50% of the time.[95] The most common sleep disturbances reported after a concussion are daytime sleepiness and insomnia, 50% and 25%, respectively.[96] In addition, sleep disturbance may be a prominent contributor to exacerbate comorbid features of depression, fatigue, and pain after a concussion[95] and worsen recovery because normal recuperative functions of sleep are altered.[97]

A return to baseline cognition and self-reported symptoms are key priorities that could be adopted to ensure player safety.[98,99] It has been demonstrated, however, that athletes sleeping fewer than 7 hours the previous night of testing would perform worse.[100] Considering that the decision of allowing a player back to play results from a comparison of preconcussion and postconcussion performances, a valid neurocognitive baseline is needed. In that sense, sleep should be monitored throughout the year to obtain an adequate neurocognitive performance and, therefore, a valid baseline. Moreover, the difference in symptomatic presentation after a concussion is highly divergent between male and female athletes.[101] This highlights the existing gap between the type of athletes and the consideration that should be directed toward an individualize baseline assessment to better detect the symptomology of a concussion.

Concussion, regardless of severity, is an injury to the brain, and athletes who are suspected of such an injury should be monitored carefully.[102,103]

An increase in awareness has directly led to more interest into postconcussion symptoms.[104,105] Research has specifically pointed out that the continuation of poor sleep symptoms after a concussion was a reliable predictor of prolonged recovery.[106–108] Additionally, Kostyun and colleagues[109] demonstrated that during recovery, adolescents who reported greater sleep disturbance performed worse on neurocognitive testing.

Insufficient Sleep as a Risk Factor for Injury

Athletes aim to achieve peak performance for as long as possible, given typically short careers with high stakes. An online study of adolescent students (12–18 years old) reported that students sleeping less than 8.1 hours a night were 1.7 times more likely to have had an injury than their peers who slept more than 8.1 hours.[110,111] Furthermore, the same study also indicated that for each additional grade in school, students were 1.4 times more likely to have had an injury. Taken together, insufficient sleep duration may increase the risk of injury. Additionally, the summation of years of (accumulated) sleep debt may play a role in risk injury outcomes.

Nutrition plays a fundamental role in recovery and injury prevention,[29,112–114] and nutrition and sleep have a bidirectional relationship.[115–119] There is an association between the number of hours slept and the intake of dietary nutriments categories.[117] Furthermore, individuals who have a later bedtime tend to consume a higher percentage of carbohydrates, fat, and protein than the average sleepers.[120] On the other hand, some nutriment categories may have a positive effect on sleep, such as tart cherries and kiwis, that are believed to reduce the number of awakening and increasing the sleep time.[121] Although nutritional knowledge is assumed to be high among athletes[122] data are sparse on the number of athletes who are following their diets on a regular basis, and this may be impacted by poor sleep, which influences food intake.[123]

Adolescents sleeping fewer than 8 hours per night were more likely to sustain an injury[124] compared with students sleeping greater than 8 hours. These results are in line with the conclusions of Milewski and colleagues.[111] This is interesting given that the results are replicated in a population of athletes. Additionally, Von Rosen and colleagues[124] found that the recommended intake of fruits, vegetables, and fish was not met for 20%, 39%, and 43% of their athletes, respectively. Therefore, the hypothesis of combined effect of poor sleep and a poor nutrition needs to be further explored in order to better understand the mechanisms underlying injuries in athletes.

Moreover, lack of sleep and poor sleep quality exacerbate depression and anxiety symptoms,[125] which also may increase injury risk. In a study of 958 athletes, 40.6% experienced an injury of various nature.[126] At preseason, 28.8% of the 958 enrolled athletes in this study reported anxiety symptoms and 21.7% reported depressive symptoms. Those with anxiety symptoms were 2.3 times more likely to have had an injury.[126] Given the strong association between poor sleep, anxiety, and depression symptoms,[127,128] it can be speculated that insufficient sleep may indirectly lead to an injury.

Insufficient Sleep and Recovery

Poor sleep quality and sleep deprivation impair brain functions that affect a wide array of cognitive functions,[129] which may directly or indirectly facilitate recovery from mental effort and/or physical injury. Furthermore, sleep-deprived individuals might increase their intake of unhealthy foods, which ultimately impairs glycogen repletion and protein synthesis,[130] which are critical for recovery in athletes. Additionally, impaired sleep directly affects growth hormone release and alters cortisol secretion,[67] having an impact on recovery from exercise and stress. Sleep deprivation also increases proinflammatory cytokines, such as interleukin 6 and C-reactive protein levels, which are pain-facilitating agents,[131] ultimately affecting the immune system; hinders muscle recovery and repair from damages sustained in high-intensity training; and leads toward an imbalance of the autonomic nervous system.[132,133] Moreover, athletes who feel the need to push the boundaries of their capabilities may tend to develop poor sleep patterns, increasing their chances of illness (ie, medical symptoms), and this has an impact on their performance and recovery.[84]

IMPACT OF SLEEP ON MENTAL AND COGNITIVE PERFORMANCE
Vigilance and Reaction Time

Sleep restriction has been demonstrated to have a negative impact on attention and reaction times.[134–137] Furthermore, it has been demonstrated that reaction times are adversely impacted after only a 1-night, complete sleep deprivation.[74]

Sleep extension, conversely, has been shown to improve reaction times by 15% and also improve objective daytime sleepiness,[138] in a study of student athletes. Mah and colleagues,[139] extended the sleep of a college basketball team during a 5-week to 7-week period. The average total sleep time increased from 7.50 hours to 10.25 hours of sleep over this period. Student athletes improved

their reaction time scores ($P<.001$) in morning and evening testing sessions. Given that athletes often experience at least mild sleep restriction (especially during intense periods of training or competition), sleep management becomes a priority to maximize reaction time. Consistent with the findings on sleep extension, there is evidence that sleep can be banked in order to optimize vigilance and reaction time.[140–142]

Executive Function and Decision Making

Executive functions are one of the cornerstones of athletic performance.[143,144] These include the highest levels of thinking required to engineer a strategy, make a fast decision, demonstrate cognitive flexibility, and manage the prioritization of attention. Deep sleep/slow wave sleep seems to have different restorative functions both at the neurophysiologic and phenomenological levels. Deep sleep seems to have a beneficial impact on the prefrontal cortex, which also has a positive impact on the functions directed by this cerebral region.[145,146] Prioritization or inhibitory control ensures the control of the athlete's concentration, attention, and thoughts and suppresses the cognitive and behavioral external and internal distractions.[147,148] Cognitive flexibility is vital for athletes by ensuring efficiency and adaptation in changing tasks.[147,149] Adaptation is key in athletics; it prevents athletes from making a bad or a risky decision, and this inhibitory control is highly linked to sleep deprivation.[150,151]

These studies underscore the deleterious effects of lack of sleep on executive functions. Too little sleep may alter an athlete's ability to make a good decision versus a risky one in a split second, during the course of a game or event. Caffeine has been suggested as a countermeasure to protect against effects on risk taking or poor decision making.[152] It has been demonstrated, however, that caffeine does not replace a proper night of sleep for these functions.[75,153–155]

Learning and Memory

Learning new skills is crucial for every athlete. The roots of memory consolidations are found in sleep.[72,156–158] The ability to recall information[159] is inevitably of interest for athletes. For example, the NFL requires emphasis on the playbook, and the ability to recall complex plays is essential for participation in football. Moreover, learning and improving a motor skill are known to continue 24 hours after training.[160] In healthy young adults, non–rapid eye movement (NREM) stage 2 sleep typically represents approximately 45% to 55% of total sleep time.[161] It has been demonstrated that the duration of sleep stage 2 (NREM) is strongly correlated with the consolidation of motor skills.[162–164] Arguably, the sleep period following learning a new skill is crucial, and it has been shown that sleep restriction can have an adverse impact on the memory consolidation.[165]

Although it is true to a certain point that practice makes perfect, the results of several studies indicated that sleep after learning improves performance significantly, relative to sleep deprivation.[166–168] So perhaps sleep makes perfect. Also, sleep restriction also has a negative impact on the academic performance of student athletes.[169] 56 students were either assigned to a 5 hours' or 9 hours' time in bed for 14 consecutive days, in which participants had to study for the Graduate Record Examination. Results showed that the sleep-restricted group were significantly impacted for the recall of massed item, which is fundamental in academic success.

Another group of elite athletes, student athletes, need to be prepared not only for their competitions but also for academics. Turner and colleagues[26] found that general sleep difficulty, initial insomnia, daytime tiredness, daytime sleepiness, and insufficient sleep all were associated with decreased academic performance among student athletes. It is partially a coach's responsibility to mentor the student athletes to be ready for any kind of test, either athletic or academic. Ultimately, assessing sleep on a regular basis could provide crucial information for the coaching members and the athletes.[170] Furthermore, having a clear idea of how an athlete sleeps may help a team medical specialist prevent injuries, such as concussion.[10]

Creativity and Thinking

Through sleep, the consolidation theory suggests that learning and memory consolidation benefit creativity.[171] The relationship between sleep and creativity stems from the direct influence of sleep on learning and formation of new concepts, ideas, solutions, and, ultimately, the genesis of creativity.[172] It was demonstrated that rapid eye movement (REM) sleep can improve creative problem-solving.[173] REM sleep, according to Cai and colleagues,[173] enhanced creativity for items that are primed before sleep by more than 40%. Another study showed that stage 1 sleep was associated with fluency and flexibility, and slow wave sleep and REM sleep were associated with originality and global measure of figural creativity.[174] Furthermore, in a Remote Associates Test study, participants were faced with different levels of difficulty and the unsolved problems were presented again after a period of sufficient sleep, wake, or no delay.[175] The sleep group solved a greater number of difficult Remote Associates Test items than the other groups. These findings suggest that sleep facilitates creative thinking for harder problems. Creative problem-solving is essential for elite athletes. During every game and every competition, elite athletes are faced with decisions that either can improve or lessen their chances of winning. Therefore, it is essential to investigate how sleep can enhance problem-solving within an environment filled with distractions, coupled with the rapidity of execution, which is more typical for elite athletes than non-athletes.

IMPACT OF SLEEP ON MENTAL HEALTH

Previous studies have pointed out the bidirectional associations between sleep, daily stressors, and poor mood states.[176,177] Moreover, poor sleep quality and short sleep duration were significantly associated with cognitive interferences related to stress the next day, such as the experience of intrusive, unwanted, off-task, and potentially ruminated thoughts.[128] Additionally, associations in the opposite direction were found, such as stressful and cognitive interferences throughout the day, that would lead to an earlier bedtime and earlier wake time.[128]

Prevalence of anxiety symptoms in adult athletes ranges from 7.1% to 26%.[178,179] Student athletes report higher rates of anxiety, up to 37%.[126,180] In a study by Lastella and colleageus,[181,182] 21% of the athletes reported that anxiety was the primary reason for their awakening during the night. Additionally, Savis and colleagues,[183] reported, among student athletes, a lower sleep quality the night before a competition. Student athletes reported that the primary reason for their sleep difficulty was anxiety and that this greatly affected their performance the following day.[128,184,185] Moreover, Davenne[186] reported that continuously being in a new sleep environment exacerbated the anxiety, thus having a negative impact on sleep and therefore performance.

Athletes not getting sufficient sleep consistently show higher rates of anxiety, leading to increased difficulty in coping with new environmental challenges and stressors, a key component of performance for every athlete.[184,185] Further studies are needed to clarify this bidirectional relation in athletes in order to develop appropriate plans of action and adaptative strategies to optimize performance.

INTERVENTIONS AT THE TEAM LEVEL
Promoting a Culture of Healthy Sleep

Prioritizing sleep in athletes' preparation and recovery routines is not an easy task. There is an omnipresent attitude in society toward sleep that has been put forward where being able to tolerate insufficient sleep is a sign of mental strength and a badge of honor.[187] This attitude may influence young elite athletes who are trying to reach the highest-level performance in their respective sports. To counter this, teams can promote a culture of healthy sleep as a performance enhancer. This includes embracing the idea that sleep is essential to athletic performance and recovery and counteract the perception that getting sufficient sleep should produce a feeling of guilt. Several high-profile athletes have now publicly discussed the importance of sleep in their preparation and recovery.[188] Unfortunately, these athletes' habits are not yet the norm and, throughout the sports literature and culture, sleep is not yet a priority among elite athletes and professional team sports, although this may be changing.

Systematically Screening for Sleep Problems

Systematically screening for sleep problems is required to understand the scope of a problem, identify areas that need improvement, and identify individuals at risk for sleep problems.[18] Ideally, teams need to screen athletes at the beginning of a season and follow-up with prospective sleep assessment. Challenges include integrating sleep assessments into existing programs, decisions about what tools to use, implementing sleep assessment at multiple timepoints, and strategies for assessing sleep disorders. In addition, developing collaborative relationships with sleep providers should be a priority.[189,190]

To date, only 1 sleep questionnaire has been validated in athletes, the ASSQ.[45] Another promising tool is the Athlete Sleep Behavioral Questionnaire,[191] which addresses mainly poor sleep behavior.

Treating Sleep Disorders

In order to treat sleep disorders among elite athletes, proper sleep screening is essential. Different types of athletes may be differently susceptible to certain types of sleep disorders. For example, American football players may have a higher prevalence of sleep apnea due to their physical attributes,[192,193] and swimmers may experience circadian rhythm problems due to their early practice schedules.[42]

Sports medicine teams should be educated on diagnosing and treating sleep disorders and referring to sleep specialists when appropriate,[194] and education about sleep disorders should be provided to both athletes and staff.[18] Furthermore, the sports medicine specialist also should be the provider and the promoter of good sleep behavior and its beneficial effects on athletic and academic performance.

When sleep disorders are identified, appropriate evidence-based treatments should be applied, just as in nonathletes,[11,18] including positive airway pressure therapy and oral appliances for sleep apnea and cognitive behavioral therapy for insomnia. Sometimes, however, evidence-based treatments of sleep disorders in athletes can be problematic. For example, sedating medications may be clinically indicated but may impede athletic performance, and some empirically supported treatments actually may be banned substances in sport.[11] For this reason, clinical providers may need to be sensitive to these issues and may need to consider whether sedating treatments impair performance or whether stimulating treatments are restricted because they are performance enhancing.

Managing Training and Travel Schedules

The relationship between training loads, timing, intensity, sleep, and performance is likely complex and not entirely understood. An increase in training load and training intensity, and decrease in hours of sleep, is associated with increased injury risk.[195] Therefore, training more efficiently may be preferable to training longer or harder. This would be more preferable to the accumulation of training load without a profitable recovery, accompanied by a decrease in performance and need for an extended period of recovery.[196,197]

SUMMARY AND FUTURE DIRECTIONS

Sleep health is an important consideration for athletic performance. Athletes are at high risk of insufficient sleep duration (ie, less than 7–8 hours per night), poor sleep quality (eg, difficulty initiating or maintaining sleep or other sleep difficulties), daytime sleepiness and fatigue, suboptimal sleep schedules (eg, too early or too late), irregular sleep schedules, and sleep and circadian disorders (especially insomnia and sleep apnea). These issues, individually and in combination, likely have an impact on athletic performance via several domains. Sleep loss and/or poor sleep quality can impair muscular strength, speed, and other aspects of physical performance. Sleep issues also can increase risk of concussions and other injuries and impair recovery after injury. Cognitive performance is also impacted in several domains, including vigilance, learning and memory, decision-making, and creativity. Sleep also plays important roles in mental health, which is

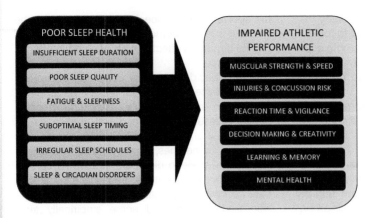

Fig. 1. Relationships between sleep health and athletic performance.

important not only for athletic performance but also the well-being of athletes in general. **Fig. 1** depicts a summary of these findings. These relationships have begun to be formally incorporated into athletics organizations, with official position statements that address sleep health published by the NCAA and the IOC.[11,18]

Much future research on sleep in athletes is needed. This is because athletes represent a diverse group of individuals, and most studies in athletes are small, confined to a single team and/or sport, and include inconsistent measurement approaches. In particular, it is not clear what the best strategy is for assessing sleep parameters in athletes, and it likely may depend on factors intrinsic to the sport or activity. Additionally, it is not known if standard approaches should be adapted. There also is a lack of trials of sleep interventions thought to have a positive impact on sleep and still an insufficient number of studies describing how improving sleep can improve performance. Despite that, there is a large and growing body of evidence that clearly establishes sleep health as an important factor in sport.

Improving sleep in athletes through sleep education at every level of sports organizations has significant implications for health, athletic performance, academic performance, and beyond, given the influence each athlete has on the general population as a role model. This not only will provide an opportunity to explore a crucial aspect of mental and physical health but also pave the way for new interventions in the area of mental well-being. Tracking sleep through questionnaires, wearables, and other objective devices is promising but there still are a lot of question marks remaining. It is, therefore, crucial to develop strategies to mitigate sleep difficulties, not only for physical performance but also for mental well-being, which will require additional data for a better understanding of the science of sleep.

DISCLOSURE

Dr M.A. Grandner has received grants from Jazz Pharmaceuticals, National Institutes of Health, Nexalin Technology, and Kemin Foods. He has performed consulting activities for Fitbit, Natrol, Casper, Curaegis, Thrive, Pharmavite, SPV, Night-Food, and Merck. This work was supported by R01MD011600 and an Innovation Grant from the National Collegiate Athletics Association.

REFERENCES

1. Lucidi F, Lombardo C, Russo PM, et al. Sleep complaints in Italian Olympic and recreational athletes. J Clin Sport Psychol 2007;1(2):121–9.
2. Samuels C. Sleep, recovery, and performance: the new frontier in high-performance athletics. Neurol Clin 2008;26(1):169–80.
3. Swinbourne R, Gill N, Vaile J, et al. Prevalence of poor sleep quality, sleepiness and obstructive sleep apnea risk factors in athletes. Eur J Sport Sci 2016;16(7):850–8.
4. Leeder J, Glaister M, Pizzoferro K, et al. Sleep duration and quality in elite athletes measured using wristwatch actigraphy. J Sports Sci 2012; 30(6):541–5.
5. Bleyer F, Barbosa D, Andrade R, et al. Sleep and musculoskeletal complaints among elite athletes of Santa Catarina. Rev dor São Paulo 2015;16(2): 102–8.
6. Bonnet MH, Arand DL. Hyperarousal and insomnia: state of the science. Sleep Med Rev 2010;14(1):9–15.
7. Tsunoda K, Hotta K, Mutsuzaki H, et al. Sleep status in male wheelchair basketball players on a Japanese national team. J Sleep Disord Ther 2015; 4(4):1–4.
8. George CF, Kab V, Kab P, et al. Sleep and breathing in professional football players. Sleep Med 2003;4(4):317–25.
9. Albuquerque FN, Kuniyoshi FHS, Calvin AD, et al. Sleep-disordered breathing, hypertension, and

obesity in retired National Football League players. J Am Coll Cardiol 2010;56(17):1432–3.

10. Raikes AC, Athey A, Alfonso-Miller P, et al. Insomnia and daytime sleepiness: risk factors for sports-related concussion. Sleep Med 2019;58:66–74.

11. Reardon CL, Hainline B, Aron CM, et al. Mental health in elite athletes: international Olympic Committee consensus statement (2019). Br J Sports Med 2019;53(11):667–99.

12. Reilly T, Waterhouse J. Sport, exercise and environmental physiology. Edinburgh: Elsevier; 2005. p. 89–115.

13. NCAA. The student-athlete perspective of the college experience findings from the NCAA GOALS and SCORE studies. 2008. Available at: https://www.ncaa.org/sites/default/files/The%20Student Athlete%20Perspective%20of%20the%20College%20Experience.pdf.

14. NCAA. Defining countable athletically related activities. 2009. Available at: https://www.ncaa.org/sites/default/files/Charts.pdf.

15. NCAA. How student-athletes feel about time demands. 2017. Available at: https://www.ncaa.org/sites/default/files/2017GOALS_Time_demands_201 70628.pdf.

16. NCAA. NCAA sports sponshirship and participation rates report. 2018. Available at: https://ncaaorg.s3.amazonaws.com/research/sportpart/Oct2018RES_2017-18SportsSponsorshipParticipationRatesReport.pdf.

17. Nixdorf I, Frank R, Hautzinger M, et al. Prevalence of depressive symptoms and correlating variables among German elite athletes. J Clin Sport Psychol 2013;7(4):313–26.

18. Kroshus E, Wagner J, Wyrick D, et al. Wake up call for collegiate athlete sleep: narrative review and consensus recommendations from the NCAA Inter-association Task Force on Sleep and Wellness. British journal of sports medicine 2019;53(12): 731–6.

19. Chase JD, Roberson PA, Saunders MJ, et al. One night of sleep restriction following heavy exercise impairs 3-km cycling time-trial performance in the morning. Appl Physiol Nutr Metab 2017;42(9): 909–15.

20. Spiegel K, Leproult R, Van Cauter E. Impact of sleep debt on metabolic and endocrine function. Lancet 1999;354(9188):1435–9.

21. Spiegel K, Leproult R, L'Hermite-Baleriaux M, et al. Leptin levels are dependent on sleep duration: relationships with sympathovagal balance, carbohydrate regulation, cortisol, and thyrotropin. J Clin Endocrinol Metab 2004;89(11):5762–71.

22. Lastella M, Roach GD, Halson SL, et al. Sleep/wake behaviours of elite athletes from individual and team sports. Eur J Sport Sci 2015;15(2): 94–100.

23. Sargent C, Lastella M, Halson SL, et al. The impact of training schedules on the sleep and fatigue of elite athletes. Chronobiol Int 2014;31(10): 1160–8.

24. Sargent C, Lastella M, Romyn G, et al. How well does a commercially available wearable device measure sleep in young athletes? Chronobiol Int 2018;35(6):754–8.

25. Mah CD, Kezirian EJ, Marcello BM, et al. Poor sleep quality and insufficient sleep of a collegiate student-athlete population. Sleep Health 2018; 4(3):251–7.

26. Turner RW, Vissa K, Hall C, et al. Sleep problems are associated with academic performance in a national sample of collegiate athletes. J Am Coll Health 2019;1–8.

27. Hoshikawa M, Uchida S, Hirano Y. A subjective assessment of the prevalence and factors associated with poor sleep quality amongst elite Japanese athletes. Sports Med Open 2018;4(1):10.

28. Drew M, Vlahovich N, Hughes D, et al. Prevalence of illness, poor mental health and sleep quality and low energy availability prior to the 2016 summer Olympic games. Br J Sports Med 2018;52(1): 47–53.

29. Drew MK, Vlahovich N, Hughes D, et al. A multifactorial evaluation of illness risk factors in athletes preparing for the Summer Olympic Games. J Sci Med Sport 2017;20(8):745–50.

30. Fischer D, Lombardi DA, Marucci-Wellman H, et al. Chronotypes in the US–influence of age and sex. PLoS One 2017;12(6):e0178782.

31. Silva A, Queiroz SS, Winckler C, et al. Sleep quality evaluation, chronotype, sleepiness and anxiety of Paralympic Brazilian athletes: Beijing 2008 Paralympic Games. Br J Sports Med 2012;46(2): 150–4.

32. Lastella M, Roach GD, Halson SL, et al. The chronotype of elite athletes. J Hum Kinet 2016;54(1): 219–25.

33. Lastella M, Roach GD, Hurem DC, et al. Does chronotype affect elite athletes' capacity to cope with the training demands of elite triathlon?. In: Sargent C, Darwent D, Roach GD, editors. Living in a 24/7 world: The impact of circadian disruption on sleep. Adelaide: Australasian Chronobiology Society Press; 2018. p. 25–8.

34. Drust B, Waterhouse J, Atkinson G, et al. Circadian rhythms in sports performance—an update. Chronobiol Int 2005;22(1):21–44.

35. Beersma DG, Gordijn MC. Circadian control of the sleep–wake cycle. Physiol Behav 2007;90(2–3): 190–5.

36. Reilly T, Edwards B. Altered sleep–wake cycles and physical performance in athletes. Physiol Behav 2007;90(2–3):274–84.

37. Lack LC, Wright HR. Chronobiology of sleep in humans. Cell Mol Life Sci 2007;64(10):1205.

38. Lastella M, Roach GD, Halson SL, et al. Sleep/wake behaviour of endurance cyclists before and during competition. J Sports Sci 2015;33(3):293–9.

39. Gupta L, Morgan K, Gilchrist S. Does elite sport degrade sleep quality? A systematic review. Sports Med 2017;47(7):1317–33.

40. Samuels C, James L, Lawson D, et al. The Athlete Sleep Screening Questionnaire: a new tool for assessing and managing sleep in elite athletes. Br J Sports Med 2016;50(7):418–22.

41. Collette R, Kellmann M, Ferrauti A, et al. Relation between training load and recovery-stress state in high-performance swimming. Front Physiol 2018; 9:845.

42. Sargent C, Halson S, Roach GD. Sleep or swim? Early-morning training severely restricts the amount of sleep obtained by elite swimmers. Eur J Sport Sci 2014;14(sup1):S310–5.

43. Erlacher D, Ehrlenspiel F, Adegbesan OA, et al. Sleep habits in German athletes before important competitions or games. J Sports Sci 2011;29(8): 859–66.

44. Samuels CH. Jet lag and travel fatigue: a comprehensive management plan for sport medicine physicians and high-performance support teams. Clin J Sport Med 2012;22(3):268–73.

45. Bender AM, Lawson D, Werthner P, et al. The clinical validation of the athlete sleep screening questionnaire: an instrument to identify athletes that need further sleep assessment. Sports Med Open 2018;4(1):23.

46. Allen MS, Greenlees I, Jones M. Personality in sport: a comprehensive review. Int Rev Sport Exerc Psychol 2013;6(1):184–208.

47. American College Health Association. American College Health Association-National College Health Assessment, Fall 2015, Spring 2016, Fall 2016, Spring 2017, Fall 2017 [data file]. Hanover (MD): American College Health Association. [producer and distributor] 2018-11-15.

48. Harvey CJ, Gehrman P, Espie CA. Who is predisposed to insomnia: a review of familial aggregation, stress-reactivity, personality and coping style. Sleep Med Rev 2014;18(3):237–47.

49. Fowler P, Duffield R, Howle K, et al. Effects of northbound long-haul international air travel on sleep quantity and subjective jet lag and wellness in professional Australian soccer players. Int J Sports Physiol Perform 2015;10(5):648–54.

50. Fowler PM, Duffield R, Lu D, et al. Effects of long-haul transmeridian travel on subjective jet-lag and self-reported sleep and upper respiratory symptoms in professional rugby league players. Int J Sports Physiol Perform 2016; 11(7):876–84.

51. Dunican IC, Martin DT, Halson SL, et al. The effects of the removal of electronic devices for 48 hours on sleep in elite judo athletes. J Strength Cond Res 2017;31(10):2832–9.

52. Emsellem HA, Murtagh KE. Sleep apnea and sports performance. Clin Sports Med 2005;24(2): 329–41.

53. Ahbab S, Ataoğlu HE, Tuna M, et al. Neck circumference, metabolic syndrome and obstructive sleep apnea syndrome; evaluation of possible linkage. Med Sci Monit 2013;19:111.

54. Mihaere KM, Harris R, Gander PH, et al. Obstructive sleep apnea in New Zealand adults: prevalence and risk factors among Māori and non-Māori. Sleep 2009;32(7):949–56.

55. Rice TB, Dunn RE, Lincoln AE, et al. Sleep-disordered breathing in the National Football League. Sleep 2010;33(6):819–24.

56. Dobrosielski DA, Nichols D, Ford J, et al. Estimating the prevalence of sleep-disordered breathing among collegiate football players. Respir Care 2016;61(9):1144–50.

57. Tuomilehto H, Vuorinen VP, Penttilä E, et al. Sleep of professional athletes: underexploited potential to improve health and performance. J Sports Sci 2017;35(7):704–10.

58. Jackson ML, Howard ME, Barnes M. Cognition and daytime functioning in sleep-related breathing disorders. Brain Res 2011;190:53–68. Elsevier.

59. Fagundes SB, Fagundes DJ, Carvalho LB, et al. Prevalence of restless legs syndrome in runners. Sleep Med 2010;33:A252. One Westbrook Corporate CTR, STE 920, Westchester, IL 60154 USA: Amer Acad Sleep Medicine.

60. Dunican IC, Walsh J, Higgins CC, et al. Prevalence of sleep disorders and sleep problems in an elite super rugby union team. J Sports Sci 2019;37(8): 950–7.

61. Edwards BJ, Waterhouse J. Effects of one night of partial sleep deprivation upon diurnal rhythms of accuracy and consistency in throwing darts. Chronobiol Int 2009;26(4):756–68.

62. Horne JA, Pettitt AN. Sleep deprivation and the physiological response to exercise under steady-state conditions in untrained subjects. Sleep 1984;7(2):168–79.

63. Martin BJ. Effect of sleep deprivation on tolerance of prolonged exercise. Eur J Appl Physiol Occup Physiol 1981;47(4):345–54.

64. Mougin F, Davenne D, Simon-Rigaud ML, et al. Disturbance of sports performance after partial sleep deprivation. C R Seances Soc Biol Fil 1989; 183(5):461–6.

65. Mougin F, Simon-Rigaud ML, Davenne D, et al. Effects of sleep disturbances on subsequent physical performance. Eur J Appl Physiol Occup Physiol 1991;63(2):77–82.

66. Mougin F, Bourdin H, Simon-Rigaud ML, et al. Effects of a selective sleep deprivation on subsequent anaerobic performance. Int J Sports Med 1996;17(02):115–9.

67. Mougin F, Bourdin H, Simon-Rigaud ML, et al. Hormonal responses to exercise after partial sleep deprivation and after a hypnotic drug-induced sleep. J Sports Sci 2001;19(2):89–97.

68. Souissi N, Souissi M, Souissi H, et al. Effect of time of day and partial sleep deprivation on short-term, high-power output. Chronobiol Int 2008;25(6): 1062–76.

69. Abedelmalek S, Souissi N, Chtourou H, et al. Effects of partial sleep deprivation on proinflammatory cytokines, growth hormone, and steroid hormone concentrations during repeated brief sprint interval exercise. Chronobiol Int 2013;30(4): 502–9.

70. Souissi N, Chtourou H, Aloui A, et al. Effects of time-of-day and partial sleep deprivation on short-term maximal performances of judo competitors. J Strength Cond Res 2013;27(9): 2473–80.

71. Abbiss CR, Laursen PB. Models to explain fatigue during prolonged endurance cycling. Sports Med 2005;35(10):865–98.

72. Stickgold R. Sleep-dependent memory consolidation. Nature 2005;437(7063):1272.

73. Walker MP, Stickgold R. It's practice, with sleep, that makes perfect: implications of sleep-dependent learning and plasticity for skill performance. Clin Sports Med 2005;24(2):301–17.

74. Taheri M, Arabameri E. The effect of sleep deprivation on choice reaction time and anaerobic power of college student athletes. Asian J Sports Med 2012;3(1):15.

75. Reyner LA, Horne JA. Sleep restriction and serving accuracy in performance tennis players, and effects of caffeine. Physiol Behav 2013;120: 93–6.

76. Ben RC, Latiri I, Dogui M, et al. Effects of one-night sleep deprivation on selective attention and isometric force in adolescent karate athletes. J Sports Med Phys Fitness 2017;57(6):752–9.

77. Omisade A, Buxton OM, Rusak B. Impact of acute sleep restriction on cortisol and leptin levels in young women. Physiol Behav 2010;99(5):651–6.

78. Oliver SJ, Costa RJ, Laing SJ, et al. One night of sleep deprivation decreases treadmill endurance performance. Eur J Appl Physiol 2009;107(2): 155–61.

79. Skein M, Duffield R, Edge J, et al. Intermittent-sprint performance and muscle glycogen after 30 h of sleep deprivation. Med Sci Sports Exerc 2011;43(7):1301–11.

80. Katirji B. Clinical neurophysiology: clinical electromyography. Philadelphia: Saunders Elsevier; 2012.

81. Costill DL, Flynn MG, Kirwan JP, et al. Effects of repeated days of intensified training on muscle glycogen and swimming performance. Med Sci Sports Exerc 1988;20(3):249–54.

82. Le Meur Y, Duffield R, Skein M. Sleep. In: Hausswirth C, Mujika I, editors. Recovery for performance in sport. Champaign (IL): Human Kinetics; 2012. p. 99–107.

83. Guezennec CY, Satabin P, Legrand H, et al. Physical performance and metabolic changes induced by combined prolonged exercise and different energy intakes in humans. Eur J Appl Physiol Occup Physiol 1994;68(6):525–30.

84. Hausswirth C, Louis J, Aubry A, et al. Evidence of disturbed sleep and increased illness in over-reached endurance athletes. Med Sci Sports Exerc 2014;46(5):1036–45.

85. Jung CM, Melanson EL, Frydendall EJ, et al. Energy expenditure during sleep, sleep deprivation and sleep following sleep deprivation in adult humans. J Physiol 2011;589(1):235–44.

86. Markwald RR, Melanson EL, Smith MR, et al. Impact of insufficient sleep on total daily energy expenditure, food intake, and weight gain. Proc Natl Acad Sci U S A 2013;110(14):5695–700.

87. Waterhouse J, Atkinson G, Edwards B, et al. The role of a short post-lunch nap in improving cognitive, motor, and sprint performance in participants with partial sleep deprivation. J Sports Sci 2007; 25(14):1557–66.

88. Zhong X, Hilton HJ, Gates GJ, et al. Increased sympathetic and decreased parasympathetic cardiovascular modulation in normal humans with acute sleep deprivation. J Appl Physiol (1985) 2005;98(6):2024–32.

89. Achten J, Jeukendrup AE. Heart rate monitoring. Sports Med 2003;33(7):517–38.

90. Hynynen ESA, Uusitalo A, Konttinen N, et al. Heart rate variability during night sleep and after awakening in overtrained athletes. Med Sci Sports Exerc 2006;38(2):313.

91. Azboy O, Kaygisiz Z. Effects of sleep deprivation on cardiorespiratory functions of the runners and volleyball players during rest and exercise. Acta Physiol Hung 2009;96(1):29–36.

92. Harmon KG, Drezner JA, Gammons M, et al. American Medical Society for Sports Medicine position statement: concussion in sport. Br J Sports Med 2013;47(1):15–26.

93. Depadilla L, Miller GF, Jones SE, et al. Self-reported concussions from playing a sport or being physically active among high school students—United States, 2017. MMWR Morb Mortal Wkly Rep 2018;67(24):682.

94. Rivara FP, Schiff MA, Chrisman SP, et al. The effect of coach education on reporting of concussions among high school athletes after passage of a

concussion law. Am J Sports Med 2014;42(5): 1197–203.

95. Mathias JL, Alvaro PK. Prevalence of sleep disturbances, disorders, and problems following traumatic brain injury: a meta-analysis. Sleep Med 2012;13(7):898–905.

96. Verma A, Anand V, Verma NP. Sleep disorders in chronic traumatic brain injury. J Clin Sleep Med 2007;3(04):357–62.

97. Weber M, Webb CA, Killgore WDS. A brief and selective review of treatment approaches for sleep disturbance following traumatic brain injury. J Sleep Disord Ther 2013;2:110.

98. McCrory P, Meeuwisse WH, Aubry M, et al. Consensus statement on concussion in sport—the 4th International Conference on Concussion in sport held in Zurich, November 2012. PM R 2013; 5(4):255–79.

99. McCrory P, Meeuwisse W, Dvorak J, et al. Consensus statement on concussion in sport—the 5th international conference on concussion in sport held in Berlin, October 2016. Br J Sports Med 2017;51(11):838–47.

100. McClure DJ, Zuckerman SL, Kutscher SJ, et al. Baseline neurocognitive testing in sports-related concussions: the importance of a prior night's sleep. Am J Sports Med 2014;42(2):472–8.

101. Brown DA, Elsass JA, Miller AJ, et al. Differences in symptom reporting between males and females at baseline and after a sports-related concussion: a systematic review and meta-analysis. Sports Med 2015;45(7):1027–40.

102. Graham R, Rivara FP, Ford MA, et al. Sports-related concussion in youth: Improving the science, changing the culture. Washington, DC: The National Acadamies Press; 2014.

103. McCrory P, Meeuwisse WH, Echemendia RJ, et al. What is the lowest threshold to make a diagnosis of concussion? Br J Sports Med 2013;47(5):268–71.

104. Eisenberg MA, Meehan WP, Mannix R. Duration and course of post-concussive symptoms. Pediatrics 2014;133(6):999–1006.

105. Lau BC, Collins MW, Lovell MR. Cutoff scores in neurocognitive testing and symptom clusters that predict protracted recovery from concussions in high school athletes. Neurosurgery 2011;70(2): 371–9.

106. Gosselin N, Lassonde M, Petit D, et al. Sleep following sport-related concussions. Sleep Med 2009;10(1):35–46.

107. Lau BC, Collins MW, Lovell MR. Sensitivity and specificity of subacute computerized neurocognitive testing and symptom evaluation in predicting outcomes after sports-related concussion. Am J Sports Med 2011;39(6):1209–16.

108. Sufrinko AM, Howie EK, Elbin RJ, et al. A preliminary investigation of accelerometer-derived sleep and physical activity following sport-related concussion. J Head Trauma Rehabil 2018;33(5):E64–74.

109. Kostyun RO, Milewski MD, Hafeez I. Sleep disturbance and neurocognitive function during the recovery from a sport-related concussion in adolescents. Am J Sports Med 2015;43(3):633–40.

110. Jones C, Griffiths P, Towers P, et al. Pre-season injury and illness associations with perceptual wellness, neuromuscular fatigue, sleep and training load in elite rugby union. Australian Journal of Strength and Conditioning; 2018.

111. Milewski MD, Skaggs DL, Bishop GA, et al. Chronic lack of sleep is associated with increased sports injuries in adolescent athletes. J Pediatr Orthop 2014;34(2):129–33.

112. Mountjoy M, Sundgot-Borgen JK, Burke LM, et al. IOC consensus statement on relative energy deficiency in sport (RED-S): 2018 update. Br J Sports Med 2018;52(11):687–97.

113. Smyth EA, Newman P, Waddington G, et al. Injury prevention strategies specific to pre-elite athletes competing in Olympic and professional sports - A systematic review. J Sci Med Sport 2019;22(8): 887–901.

114. Pyne DB, Verhagen EA, Mountjoy M. Nutrition, illness, and injury in aquatic sports. Int J Sport Nutr Exerc Metab 2014;24(4):460–9.

115. Chaput JP, Dutil C. Lack of sleep as a contributor to obesity in adolescents: impacts on eating and activity behaviors. Int J Behav Nutr Phys Act 2016; 13(1):103.

116. Grandner MA, Jackson N, Gerstner JR, et al. Dietary nutrients associated with short and long sleep duration. Data from a nationally representative sample. Appetite 2013;64:71–80.

117. Grandner MA, Jackson N, Gerstner JR, et al. Sleep symptoms associated with intake of specific dietary nutrients. J Sleep Res 2014;23(1):22–34.

118. Halson SL. Monitoring training load to understand fatigue in athletes. Sports Med 2014;44(2):139–47.

119. Ordóñez FM, Oliver AJS, Bastos PC, et al. Sleep improvement in athletes: use of nutritional supplements. Am J Sports Med 2017;34:93–9.

120. Baron KG, Reid KJ, Van Horn L, et al. Contribution of evening macronutrient intake to total caloric intake and body mass index. Appetite 2013;60: 246–51.

121. Lin HH, Tsai PS, Fang SC, et al. Effect of kiwifruit consumption on sleep quality in adults with sleep problems. Asia Pac J Clin Nutr 2011;20(2):169.

122. Heaney S, O'Connor H, Michael S, et al. Nutrition knowledge in athletes: a systematic review. Int J Sport Nutr Exerc Metab 2011;21(3):248–61.

123. Shechter A, Grandner MA, St-Onge MP. The role of sleep in the control of food intake. Am J Lifestyle Med 2014;8(6):371–4.

124. Von Rosen P, Frohm A, Kottorp A, et al. Too little sleep and an unhealthy diet could increase the risk of sustaining a new injury in adolescent elite athletes. Scand J Med Sci Sports 2017;27(11): 1364–71.

125. Owens J, Adolescent Sleep Working Group. Insufficient sleep in adolescents and young adults: an update on causes and consequences. Pediatrics 2014;134(3):e921–32.

126. Li H, Moreland JJ, Peek-Asa C, et al. Preseason anxiety and depressive symptoms and prospective injury risk in collegiate athletes. Am J Sports Med 2017;45(9):2148–55.

127. Baglioni C, Battagliese G, Feige B, et al. Insomnia as a predictor of depression: a meta-analytic evaluation of longitudinal epidemiological studies. J Affect Disord 2011;135(1–3):10–9.

128. Lee S, Buxton OM, Andel R, et al. Bidirectional associations of sleep with cognitive interference in employees' work days. Sleep Health 2019;5(3): 298–308.

129. Killgore WD. Effects of sleep deprivation on cognition. Prog Brain Res 2010;185:105–29. Elsevier.

130. Morselli L, Leproult R, Balbo M, et al. Role of sleep duration in the regulation of glucose metabolism and appetite. Best Pract Res Clin Endocrinol Metab 2010;24(5):687–702.

131. McMahon SB, Cafferty WB, Marchand F. Immune and glial cell factors as pain mediators and modulators. Experimental neurology 2005;192(2): 444–62.

132. Haack M, Sanchez E, Mullington JM. Elevated inflammatory markers in response to prolonged sleep restriction are associated with increased pain experience in healthy volunteers. Sleep 2007;30(9):1145–52.

133. Haack M, Lee E, Cohen DA, et al. Activation of the prostaglandin system in response to sleep loss in healthy humans: potential mediator of increased spontaneous pain. Pain 2009;145(1–2):136–41.

134. Basner M, Dinges DF. Maximizing sensitivity of the psychomotor vigilance test (PVT) to sleep loss. Sleep 2011;34(5):581–91.

135. Dinges DF, Pack F, Williams K, et al. Cumulative sleepiness, mood disturbance, and psychomotor vigilance performance decrements during a week of sleep restricted to 4–5 hours per night. Sleep 1997;20(4):267–77.

136. Włodarczyk D, Jaśkowski P, Nowik A. Influence of sleep deprivation and auditory intensity on reaction time and response force. Percept Mot Skills 2002; 94(3_suppl):1101–12.

137. Wolanin A, Hong E, Marks D, et al. Prevalence of clinically elevated depressive symptoms in college athletes and differences by gender and sport. Br J Sports Med 2016;50(3):167–71.

138. Kamdar BB, Kaplan KA, Kezirian EJ, et al. The impact of extended sleep on daytime alertness, vigilance, and mood. Sleep Med 2004;5(5): 441–8.

139. Mah CD, Mah KE, Kezirian EJ, et al. The effects of sleep extension on the athletic performance of collegiate basketball players. Sleep 2011;34(7): 943–50.

140. Arnal PJ, Sauvet F, Leger D, et al. Benefits of sleep extension on sustained attention and sleep pressure before and during total sleep deprivation and recovery. Sleep 2015;38(12):1935–43.

141. Arnal PJ, Lapole T, Erblang M, et al. Sleep extension before sleep loss: effects on performance and neuromuscular function. Med Sci Sports Exerc 2016;48(8):1595–603.

142. Rupp TL, Wesensten NJ, Bliese PD, et al. Banking sleep: realization of benefits during subsequent sleep restriction and recovery. Sleep 2009;32(3): 311–21.

143. Marchetti R, Forte R, Borzacchini M, et al. Physical and motor fitness, sport skills and executive function in adolescents: a moderated prediction model. Psychology 2015;6(14):1915.

144. Micai M, Kavussanu M, Ring C. Executive function is associated with antisocial behavior and aggression in athletes. J Sport Exerc Psychol 2015;37(5): 469–76.

145. Goel N, Rao H, Durmer JS, et al. Neurocognitive consequences of sleep deprivation. Semin Neurol 2009;29(04):320–39. © Thieme Medical Publishers.

146. Wilckens KA, Erickson KI, Wheeler ME. Age-related decline in controlled retrieval: the role of the PFC and sleep. Neural Plast 2012;2012: 624795.

147. Diamond A. Executive functions. Annu Rev Psychol 2013;64:135–68.

148. Lehto JE, Juujärvi P, Kooistra L, et al. Dimensions of executive functioning: evidence from children. Br J Dev Psychol 2003;21(1):59–80.

149. Kiesel A, Steinhauser M, Wendt M, et al. Control and interference in task switching—A review. Psychol Bull 2010;136(5):849.

150. Killgore WD, Balkin TJ, Wesensten NJ. Impaired decision making following 49 h of sleep deprivation. J Sleep Res 2006;15(1):7–13.

151. Rossa KR, Smith SS, Allan AC, et al. The effects of sleep restriction on executive inhibitory control and affect in young adults. J Adolesc Health 2014; 55(2):287–92.

152. Killgore WD, Kamimori GH, Balkin TJ. Caffeine protects against increased risk-taking propensity during severe sleep deprivation. J Sleep Res 2011; 20(3):395–403.

153. Clark I, Landolt HP. Coffee, caffeine, and sleep: a systematic review of epidemiological studies and

randomized controlled trials. Sleep Med Rev 2017; 31:70–8.

154. Drake C, Roehrs T, Shambroom J, et al. Caffeine effects on sleep taken 0, 3, or 6 hours before going to bed. J Clin Sleep Med 2013;9(11):1195–200.

155. Dunican IC, Higgins CC, Jones MJ, et al. Caffeine use in a super rugby game and its relationship to post-game sleep. Eur J Sport Sci 2018;18(4): 513–23.

156. Huber R, Ghilardi MF, Massimini M, et al. Local sleep and learning. Nature 2004;430(6995):78.

157. Maquet P. The role of sleep in learning and memory. Science 2001;294(5544):1048–52.

158. Stickgold R, Hobson JA, Fosse R, et al. Sleep, learning, and dreams: off-line memory reprocessing. Science 2001;294(5544):1052–7.

159. Gais S, Lucas B, Born J. Sleep after learning aids memory recall. Learn Mem 2006;13(3):259–62.

160. Karni A, Meyer G, Rey-Hipolito C, et al. The acquisition of skilled motor performance: fast and slow experience-driven changes in primary motor cortex. Proc Natl Acad Sci U S A 1998;95(3):861–8.

161. Carskadon MA, Dement WC. Normal human sleep: an overview. In: Kryger MH, Roth T, Dement WC, editors. Principles and practice of sleep medicine. St Louis (MO): Saunders/Elsevier; 2011. p. 16–26.

162. Albouy G, King BR, Maquet P, et al. Hippocampus and striatum: dynamics and interaction during acquisition and sleep-related motor sequence memory consolidation. Hippocampus 2013; 23(11):985–1004.

163. Doyon J, Gabitov E, Vahdat S, et al. Current issues related to motor sequence learning in humans. Curr Opin Behav Sci 2018;20:89–97.

164. Walker MP, Brakefield T, Morgan A, et al. Practice with sleep makes perfect: sleep-dependent motor skill learning. Neuron 2002;35(1):205–11.

165. Curcio G, Ferrara M, De Gennaro L. Sleep loss, learning capacity and academic performance. Sleep Med Rev 2006;10(5):323–37.

166. Albouy G, Vandewalle G, Sterpenich V, et al. Sleep stabilizes visuomotor adaptation memory: a functional magnetic resonance imaging study. J Sleep Res 2013;22(2):144–54.

167. Ashworth A, Hill CM, Karmiloff-Smith A, et al. Sleep enhances memory consolidation in children. J Sleep Res 2014;23(3):304–10.

168. Walker MP, Stickgold R. Sleep, memory, and plasticity. Annu Rev Psychol 2006;57:139–66.

169. Huang S, Deshpande A, Yeo SC, et al. Sleep restriction impairs vocabulary learning when adolescents cram for exams: the need for sleep study. Sleep 2016;39(9):1681–90.

170. Okano K, Kaczmaryk J, Dave N, et al. Sleep quality, duration, and consistency are associated with better academic performance in college students. NPJ Sci Learn 2019;4(1):16.

171. Oudiette D, Constantinescu I, Leclair-Visonneau L, et al. Evidence for the re-enactment of a recently learned behavior during sleepwalking. PLoS One 2011;6(3):e18056.

172. Marguilho R, Jesus SN, Viseu J, et al. Sleep and creativity: a quantitative review. In: Milcu M, Krall H, Dan P, editors. Prospecting interdisciplinarity in health, education and social sciences. Bucharest: Editura Universitara; 2014. p. 117–26.

173. Cai DJ, Mednick SA, Harrison EM, et al. REM, not incubation, improves creativity by priming associative networks. Proc Natl Acad Sci U S A 2009; 106(25):10130–4.

174. Drago V, Foster PS, Heilman KM, et al. Cyclic alternating pattern in sleep and its relationship to creativity. Sleep Med 2011;12(4):361–6.

175. Sio UN, Monaghan P, Ormerod T. Sleep on it, but only if it is difficult: effects of sleep on problem solving. Mem Cognit 2013;41(2):159–66.

176. Lee S, Crain TL, McHale SM, et al. Daily antecedents and consequences of nightly sleep. J Sleep Res 2017;26(4):498–509.

177. Sin NL, Almeida DM, Crain TL, et al. Bidirectional, temporal associations of sleep with positive events, affect, and stressors in daily life across a week. Ann Behav Med 2017;51(3):402–15.

178. Gouttebarge V, Frings-Dresen MHW, Sluiter JK. Mental and psychosocial health among current and former professional footballers. Occup Med 2015;65(3):190–6.

179. Gulliver A, Griffiths KM, Mackinnon A, et al. The mental health of Australian elite athletes. J Sci Med Sport 2015;18(3):255–61.

180. Storch EA, Storch JB, Killiany EM, et al. Self-reported psychopathology in athletes: a comparison of intercollegiate student-athletes and non-athletes. J Sport Behav 2005;28(1):86–97.

181. Lastella M, Lovell GP, Sargent C. Athletes' precompetitive sleep behaviour and its relationship with subsequent precompetitive mood and performance. Eur J Sport Sci 2014;14(sup1): S123–30.

182. Lastella M, Roach GD, Halson SL, et al. The effects of transmeridian travel and altitude on sleep: preparation for football competition. J Sports Sci Med 2014;13(3):718.

183. Savis JC, Eliot JF, Gansneder B, et al. A subjective means of assessing college athletes' sleep: a modification of the morningness/eveningness questionnaire. Int J Sport Psychol 1997;28(2): 157–70.

184. Brassington GS. Sleep problems. In: Mostofsky DL, Zaichkowsky LD, editors. Medical and psychological aspects of sport and exercise. Morgantown (WV): Fitness Information Technology; 2002. p. 193–204.

185. Walters PH. Sleep, the athlete, and performance. Strength Condit J 2002;24(2):17–24.

186. Davenne D. Sleep of athletes–problems and possible solutions. Biol Rhythm Res 2009;40(1):45–52.

187. Adler M. In today's world, the well-rested lose respect. Morning edition. Washington, DC: National Public Radio; 2009.

188. Schultz J. These famous athletes rely on sleep for peak performance, Huffington Post. 2014. Available at: http://www.huffingtonpost.com/2014/08/13/these-famous-athletes-rely-on-sleep_n_5659345.html. Accessed October 1, 2019.

189. Grandner MA, Alfonso-Miller P, Fernandez-Mendoza J, et al. Sleep: important considerations for the prevention of cardiovascular disease. Curr Opin Cardiol 2016;31(5):551.

190. Grandner MA. Healthy sleep for student-athletes: A guide for athletics departments and coaches. NCAA Sport Science Institute Newsletter, 4(2).

191. Driller MW, Mah CD, Halson SL. Development of the athlete sleep behavior questionnaire: a tool for identifying maladaptive sleep practices in elite athletes. Sleep Sci 2018;11(1):37.

192. George CF, Kab V. Sleep-disordered breathing in the National Football League is not a trivial matter. Sleep 2011;34(3):245.

193. Rogers AJ, Xia K, Soe K, et al. Obstructive sleep apnea among players in the National Football League: a scoping review. J Sleep Disord Ther 2017;6(5) [pii:278].

194. Brown GT, Hainline B, Kroshus E, et al. Mind, body and sport: understanding and supporting student-athlete mental wellness. Indianapolis: NCAA; 2014.

195. Von Rosen P, Frohm A, Kottorp A, et al. Multiple factors explain injury risk in adolescent elite athletes: applying a biopsychosocial perspective. Scand J Med Sci Sports 2017;27(12):2059–69.

196. Meeusen R, Duclos M, Foster C, et al. Prevention, diagnosis, and treatment of the overtraining syndrome: joint consensus statement of the European College of Sport Science and the American College of Sports Medicine. Med Sci Sports Exerc 2013;45(1):186–205.

197. Halson SL, Jeukendrup AE. Does overtraining exist? Sports medicine 2004;34(14):967–81.

Sleep Predicts Collegiate Academic Performance
Implications for Equity in Student Retention and Success

J. Roxanne Prichard, PhD

KEYWORDS

- Academic success • Sleep quality • Retention • Social determinants of health • Sleep environment

KEY POINTS

- Multiple aspects of sleep, including total sleep time, sleep schedule regularity, chronotype, and nap behavior, predict academic success.
- Sleep quality is a barometer of social capital on college campuses; ethnic, racial, and sexual majority students have better sleep, as do students without histories of trauma, harassment, disability, and adverse childhood experiences.
- Sleep intervention programs, especially those that include in-depth sleep education and cognitive behavior therapy for insomnia, are successful at improving some components of student sleep.
- Improving sleep through screening, education, and improving the social and physical environments of college residences has potential to reduce educational and health disparities.

INTRODUCTION

Mary Carskadon described sleep in adolescence as the "perfect storm" of factors that impair sleep: a biological phase delay and decreased sensitivity to the homeostatic sleep drive, coupled with zeitgebers that delay sleep and necessitate early awakening.[1] Chief among these are increased use of screen-based media[2] and early high school start times, 90% of which are out of compliance with US Centers for Disease Control and Prevention recommendations.[3] These conditions have created a generation of young adults who enter college without an embodied understanding of what it feels like to be well-rested.

This perfect storm continues to rage in college, when students face additional challenges to their sleep. Sleep measures, including weekday total sleep time (TST), sleep efficiency, sleep latency, and sleep time variability, worsen in the 3 years following high school graduation.[4] This review

describes the evidence linking poor sleep with impaired academic performance; discusses mediating environmental, behavioral, and demographic factors; and highlights examples of successful health promotion initiatives. Given that students who are traditionally minoritized on college campuses tend to have worse sleep, improving sleep health emerges as an important issue for retention, equity, and inclusion.

Normative Sleep in College Students

The general consensus is that most young adults need 7 to 9 hours of sleep a night for optimal restoration and performance.[5] However, most college students report chronic insufficient sleep. Data from the spring 2018 undergraduate reference report of the American College Health Association National College Health Assessment-IIc (ACHA-NCHA), a comprehensive health survey of 140 colleges and universities in the United States

University of St. Thomas, 2115 Summit Avenue, JRC LL56, St Paul, MN 55105, USA
E-mail address: jrprichard@stthomas.edu
Twitter: @RoxannePrichard (J.R.P.)

Sleep Med Clin 15 (2020) 59–69
https://doi.org/10.1016/j.jsmc.2019.10.003
1556-407X/20/© 2019 Elsevier Inc. All rights reserved.

(n>70,000), show that 45% of students report getting enough sleep to feel rested fewer than 3 days a week.[6] In addition more than a third identified sleep difficulties as "traumatic or very difficult to handle"; only academics and finances were ranked as more problematic.[6] In addition to insufficient sleep, college students also report excessive daytime sleepiness and poor sleep quality, with most students endorsing scores more than 5 on the Pittsburgh Sleep Quality Index (PSQI).[7-9]

Despite the widespread evidence of poor sleep among college students, only about a quarter of students report having received any health information regarding sleep from their universities.[10] Sleep ranks second to last of 19 health-related topics undergraduate students report receiving information about.[6] Thus, sleep health represents an underused area to address in health promotion.

SLEEP AND ACADEMIC PERFORMANCE

More than 23% of students identify sleep problems as impediments to their academic success, third after stress (35.3%) and anxiety (28.1%). Multiple single-institution and multi-institution cross-sectional and longitudinal studies show a positive relationship between sufficient, good-quality sleep and academic success. Taylor and colleagues[11] used a prospective sleep diary approach (n = 867) to compare unique contributions of sleep problems to grade point average (GPA), controlling for health variables, high school GPA, and standardized test scores. TST and sleep schedule inconsistency emerged as the most significant predictors of academic success after high school GPA and standardized test scores, with students sleeping less than 6 or more than 9 hours a night achieving the lowest grades. Similarly, a Portuguese study (n = 1654) found that sufficient sleep was the third most important variable in predicting grades, after previous academic achievement and class attendance.[12] In a longitudinal study of more than 3000 students, those who endorsed frequent sleep deprivation in their first year had lower GPAs, 4-year graduate rates, and development of leadership skills than those who said they were only rarely or occasionally sleep deprived.[13,14]

In addition to TST, sleep quality and more consistent sleep/wakefulness schedules have been linked to academic success. Students with higher GPAs were less likely to oversleep (n = 231)[15] and had greater sleep schedule regularity (n = 61)[16] than students with lower GPAs. A prospective semester-long study of 88 students in the same introductory chemistry class found that TST, sleep schedule regularity, and sleep quality (as measured by a Fitbit algorithm) over the semester accounted for a 25% of the variance in students' course performance. Sleep on the night before exams were not predictive of next day performance.[17] A detailed analysis of the spring 2009 ACHA-NCHA dataset (n = 55,322) found that for each additional day per week an undergraduate student reported a sleep problem (eg, daytime sleepiness, difficulty falling asleep, waking up too early), the student's cumulative GPA decreased by 0.02 and the likelihood of dropping a course increased 10%, holding all other variables (eg, demographic, health, and time use demands) constant.[10]

Experimental Studies on Sleep and Learning

Healthy sleep supports students' learning capacity. In short, sleep loss is associated with poor procedural and declarative learning, and manipulation by sleep deprivation or extension worsens or improves, respectively, performance on a variety of prefrontal cortex-dependent neurocognitive tasks.[18] Teens (n = 56) assigned to 2 weeks of 9 hours in bed outperformed those assigned to 5 hours in bed on learning GRE vocabulary words on examinations the same day, 1 day, and 5 days after studying.[19] The sleep-restricted teens also showed deterioration in mood, working memory, sustained attention, and executive function.[20] In classroom studies, actigraphy-measured sleep parameters in the week between a lecture and examination accounted for 13% of the variance in scores, with short TST and later bedtimes associated with worse performance (n = 78).[21] Sleep extension challenges for extra credit (students showing ≥8 hours of TST per night in the week leading up to an examination) increased test performance, controlling for previous performance in the class.[22]

Sleep Disorders and Academic Performance

Sleep disorders are likely underdiagnosed in the college population. Only 3.7% of undergraduates report having been diagnosed or treated in the last year for insomnia, and 2.5% for any other sleep disorder. The SLEEP-50 Questionnaire screens for those at risk for sleep disorders, including obstructive sleep apnea (OSA), insomnia, narcolepsy, circadian rhythm disorders, parasomnias, and poor sleep hygiene.[23] In a cross-sectional study of students (n = 1845), the 27% who screened positive for possible sleep disorders on this scale were significantly more likely to have GPAs less than 2.0.[24] In a prospective 3-year study using the same instrument (n = 900), the 40% of students who screened positive for sleep disturbances as first-year students had lower GPAs and retention rates over the next

2 years than those who did not.[25] A separate study found that students at high risk of OSA (5%) had twice the rate of poor academic performance of their peers.[26] Screening students for sleep disorders offers an important opportunity for addressing both the health and academic success of college students.

Chronotypes and Academic Performance

First-year college students, who often have a disproportionately number of early-morning classes, have the latest bedtimes and shortest TSTs,[7] and the impact of poor sleep on academic success is 40% more pronounced for first-year students than for the general population.[10] A survey of 500 students from 2 UK universities found that first-year students in particular endorsed excessive sleepiness and a desire to start university class times 2 hours later.[27] Students with evening chronotypes, who often need to take classes at their nonpreferred learning times, are at a distinct academic disadvantage and have reduced weekday sleep quality compared with morning types.[28–31] Changes to align school start times with teens' circadian rhythms increase objectively measured weekday TSTs[29] and improve attendance and well-being in high school students.[30] At the university level, starting the academic day 50 minutes later at the US Air Force Academy resulted in improvement in grades for classes throughout the day.[31]

Physical Health

Some of the relationship between poor sleep and reduced academic performance is likely mediated by physical health. The connection between immune dysfunction and susceptibility to contagious illness is well documented.[32] Approximately 20% of undergraduates report negative academic consequences because of acute illness and an additional 2.5% because of injury.[6] A months-long prospective actigraphy study of high school students found that those who contracted acute illnesses had shorter TST overall, as well as shorter TST in the week leading up to the illness.[33] High school and college students who report sufficient sleep also report fewer orthopedic[34] and concussion[35] sports injuries, better glucose management,[36] and higher overall physical well-being.[7,37]

SLEEP HYGIENE CONSIDERATIONS
Residential Sleep Environment

Physical elements of the sleep environment, including air, noise, and light pollution, contribute to poor sleep quality.[38] Social elements such as a neighborhood's safety, walkability, and trust in neighbors are associated with better sleep.[38,39] The sleep environment for college students is notoriously cramped, noisy, and imbued with complicated social relationships. Sexton-Radek and Hartley[40] provide a wealth of information in their informative mixed methods study on sleep in the college residences. The most common environmental disturbances to sleep were in-room noise, sunlight, hallway noise, and heat; sleep efficiency negatively correlated with scores on the Young Adult Sleep Environment Inventory. Both surveys and in-depth interviews with first-year residential students emphasized noise and complex social relationships as major impediments to sleep.[41,42] Students' preferred strategies for improving sleep (eg, watching television, using alcohol, over-the-counter or prescription drugs) were often at odds with best practices in sleep hygiene.[43]

Electronics

Widespread use of electronics at night is ubiquitous, and common practices like online assignments due at midnight tacitly promote late night electronic use in college students. Screen-based media use compromises adolescent sleep through time displacement, psychological stimulation, and light-induced delays in the circadian timing system.[44,45] Two international studies have found that more than 20% of students meet the criteria for smartphone addiction, and more than 33% report negative sleep consequences from smartphone use.[46,47] A naturalistic study of 83 college students' text message habits showed that, over the course of a week, poorer subjective sleep quality was related to increased daily social media use and receiving nighttime notifications.[48] In a detailed path analysis (n>700), Rosen and colleagues[49] showed that the connection between emotional distress and sleep problems was partially mediated via smartphone usage. Research on the effectiveness of various health promotion strategies to improve sleep via healthier screen-based media strategies is warranted.

Naps

Daytime sleep is common among college students, both inadvertently falling asleep during class (>15%)[7] as well as taking intentional naps. A detailed factor analysis (n = 450) found that 50% of students napped at least once a week, and those who napped for restoration (as opposed to emotional reasons) reported better overall quality sleep.[50] Another cross-sectional survey of 440 students found that those who napped more than 3 times a week, for longer than 2 hours, or later than 6 PM had lower sleep quality than those with healthier nap behaviors.[51] Longer and later naps can reduce sleep pressure and contribute to circadian dyssynchrony, but students tend not to attribute sleep disturbances to naps.[52]

Psychoactive Substance Use

Alcohol misuse is widespread, with more than 25% of students reporting high-risk drinking in the last 2 weeks[6] and 89% reporting secondhand harm (eg, threat of violence, disruption to sleep or studies) from someone else's alcohol use in the past 30 days.[53] In the last year, more than 20% of the undergraduate population reported taking prescription psychiatric medication, and at least half as many reported nonmedical use (NMU) of prescription medications.[6] NMU of prescription stimulants and sedatives by college students has increased since 2003, and NMU eclipses prescribed use.[54] In the 2018 ACHA-NCHA, approximately 1 in 5 students reported cannabis use in the last month,[6] a figure that is expected to increase as more states decriminalize medical and recreational cannabis. A study in Canada, where medicinal cannabis has been legal since 2001, found that, of the 11% of students who were medicinal marijuana users, 80% used it for mental health conditions not included in prescribing guidelines, 85% used it recreationally, and 14% met the criteria for cannabis use disorder.[55] Last-month use of tobacco products was about 10% for undergraduates, with e-cigarettes more commonly used than cigarettes or other forms of tobacco.[6] Given the widespread use of recreational and prescription drugs by college students, sleep hygiene discussions in this population must include the impact of such substances, all of which alter sleep neurophysiology.

Self-Medication of Fatigue and Insomnia

Substantial evidence supports widespread self-medication to both induce sleep and promote wakefulness among college students. Students with greater insomnia symptoms and/or shorter TSTs are more likely to report using tobacco,[56] energy drinks,[57,58] NMU of prescriptions drugs,[59,60] alcohol,[61] and cannabis.[62,63] Sleep disorders and substance use disorders are well documented to interact in a feed-forward system, whereby substance use disrupts sleep, and disrupted sleep promotes substance misuse.[64] A two-wave longitudinal survey (n = 171) found that 25% of students reported substance use to promote sleep at least once in the last 2 weeks.[61] Students with high PSQI scores are twice as likely to report using alcohol to get to sleep, and students who report drinking to promote sleep consume ~40% more drinks a week than those who drink for social reasons.[7] In multivariate regression studies, regular tobacco use emerges as the pharmacologic factor most predictive of both bad sleep[56,65] and academic problems.[10] Given that problematic substance use independently predicts reduced academic success, albeit on levels less than or on par with sleep disturbances,[10] it is likely that substance use partially mediates the connection between sleep and academic performance.

DEMOGRAPHIC FACTORS IN SLEEP QUALITY
Ethnicity and Discrimination

Sleep quality can serve as a barometer for social capital in a particular society. People who experience material hardships (eg, employment instability, financial problems, housing instability, food insecurity, forgone medical care), discrimination, and trauma have reduced TSTs and worse sleep quality than the general population.[66,67] Also, experiencing racial discrimination independently predicts sleep disturbance, after controlling for multiple covariates (odds ratio [OR], 1.60).[68] More than 44% of black students at primarily white institutions seeking support from counseling services (n = 1500) reported being at least moderately distressed by racial discrimination.[69] In regression analyses, the level of perceived racial discrimination accounted for 37% of the variance in the presenting problems checklist, and was associated with lower-quality sleep.[69] For American Indian college students (n = 90), sense of belongingness to the university community predicted better actigraphy-measured sleep, including TST, sleep efficiency, and global subjective sleep quality.[70] These findings underscore the need to consider the social environment as a significant predictor of sleep, especially for individuals who are minorities in the social context of the university.

Poverty and Economic Insecurity

Studies in college students support the strong associations between economic security and sleep quality. Food insecurity is widespread on college campuses, with estimates of ~40% either experiencing or being at risk for food insecurity, and is correlated with fewer days a week with sufficient sleep and greater odds of poor sleep quality (OR, 2.32).[71–76] Food-insecure students were also more likely to report high stress (OR, 4.65), and a GPA < 3.0 (OR, 1.91). Black and Latinx students[74] and students who were Pell-grant recipients or living off campus[75] were most likely to be food insecure.

Work obligations are also important mediators of sleep, well-being, and academic success. More than 60% of undergraduates work while taking classes, and, of those, 36% work 20 hours or more a week.[6] A 5-day actigraphy study of sleep in full-time working students found mean weekday TSTs less than 6 hours.[72] Barone[73] frames working students as exploiting their so-called health capital as a trade-off for economic stability. In structured interviews with 19 working students, students reported being aware of their excessive tiredness, and of the connection between sleep and health, but were resigned to prioritizing sleep last in their schedules.[73]

Gender, Sexuality, and Gender-Based Violence

Gender, gender-based violence, and sexual minority status predict multiple aspects of sleep. In the 2018 ACHA-NCHA, 35.7% of college women reported that their sleep problems were traumatic or very difficult to handle, compared with 28.5% of men,[6] and women tend to have lower sleep efficiency, longer sleep latencies, and more sleep disturbances than men.[7,9] Sexual harassment and assault are linked to 36% increased odds for reporting worse sleep[74] and greater nightmares and insomnia,[75] and, among female undergraduates, 7% report stalking, 9% report abusive relationships, and 13% report unwanted sexual touching in the last 12 months.[6] In teens, sexual minority status is associated with increased odds of very short ($\leq$5 hours) TST, and this relationship is mediated by experiences of victimization.[76]

MENTAL HEALTH

Sleep quality and mental health are intricately intertwined and bidirectional,[77,78] so chronic insufficient sleep and circadian disruption must be considered as both contributing to and a consequence of eroding mental health in college students. The uptick of mental health concerns among college students has been described as a crisis and epidemic[79]; between 2011 and 2015 there was a 53% increase in adolescent psychiatric emergency department visits.[80] This rate mirrors the increasing population of adolescents over the last decade who report insufficient sleep.[2] A UK national health survey showed that, between 2005 and 2015, the percentage of 14-year-olds reporting less than 8 hours of TST doubled, and there was ~50% increase in depression, emotional distress, and self-harm, but a decrease in hazardous substance use.[81] Among college students, there was a 22% increase between 2009 and 2018 in those reporting significant difficulties in daytime sleepiness and a 37% increase in those

describing their sleep problems as traumatic or very difficult to handle.[6] More population-level research is needed understand the unique contributions of insufficient sleep to the increase in mental distress.

Sleep disturbances are clinically relevant for both the evaluation and treatment of mental health concerns. Fragmented sleep and increased wake after sleep onset serves as a transdiagnostic imbalance in the arousal system, and alterations in delta power and rapid eye movement sleep pressure are present in most mental illnesses other than seasonal affective disorder and attention-deficit/hyperactivity disorder (ADHD).[82] Attention disorders are characterized by shorter TSTs,[83] but, because the symptoms of chronic insufficient sleep mirror ADHD, it can be difficult to dissociate the two diagnostically.[84] Fragmented sleep, sleep hallucinations, and insomnia symptoms are linked with student reports of psychosislike experiences.[85] It is unlikely that most student mental health providers include a thorough assessment of sleep behaviors on intake, although this information would be helpful for accurate diagnosis and treatment.

Depression/Anxiety

Approximately one-third of students have been diagnosed or treated by a professional in the last year for depression and/or anxiety.[6] Results from a 6-campus survey (n>7000) found that although both anxiety and depression were associated with decreased sleep quality on a variety of PSQI subscales, anxiety symptoms were uniquely associated with more sleep disruptions and sleep medication use, whereas depressive symptoms were more associated with daytime dysfunction.[9] However, the PSQI shows poor divergent validity discrimination with anxiety, depression, and perceived stress in college students.[86] A study of the spring 2011 ACHA-NCHA dataset added to the literature by including students who self-reported high levels of emotional distress but who had not yet interacted with a health care provider. Of the students reporting severe emotional distress, only 45% had received a diagnosis and 35% had received treatment from a professional in the last year.[56] Clinically relevant depression or anxiety symptoms, or comorbid symptoms, were associated with a ~1 d/wk and a ~1.5 d/wk increase, respectively, in sleep disturbances compared with nonsymptomatic students. Because daytime sleepiness predicts both severe mental distress and lower academic achievement,[87] these changes in sleep quality have important implications for academic success.

Sleep and Behavioral Health Feedback Loops

Sleep disruptions exacerbate the symptoms of mental illness,[88] and mental illnesses impair sleep.[89,90] Among college students, the most commonly reported barrier to sleep is stress,[7] and poor sleep enhances physiologic responses to stressors.[91–93] Prospective population studies show that disturbed sleep is a risk factor for onset, exacerbation, and relapse of mood disorders in adolescents,[88] and that sleep disturbances, including insomnia and insufficient sleep, predict social anxiety, substance use, loneliness, social withdrawal, depression, and suicidal thoughts,[88,94–96] which 13% of undergraduates report.[6] Two actigraphy studies have shown prospective relationships between poor sleep (sleep timing variability, short sleep, insomnia) and subsequent suicidal ideation,[97] and sleep variability was a better longitudinal predictor of suicidal ideation than depressive symptoms in students at risk for suicide.[98]

However, the converse is also true: healthy sleep is a protective mental health factor for well-being in both clinical and nonclinical populations,[99,100] and treating insomnia improves depression and anxiety symptoms.[101,102] Although students with higher levels of adverse childhood experiences (ACEs) show greater sleep impairment than their peers,[103] sleep quality mediates the relationship between ACEs and multiple measures of physical and mental health.[104] Further research is needed on the capacity of sleep to serve as a modifiable protective mental health factor in college students.

SLEEP HEALTH PROMOTION

The disconnect between students who desire information from their universities regarding sleep health (60%) and those receiving it (25%)[10] suggests room for improvement in health promotion. Unless clinicians complete additional training in sleep or behavioral sleep medicine, it is unlikely they will receive more than a few hours of education about sleep in either medical school or clinical psychology doctoral programs.[105,106] According to the 2018 Center for Collegiate Mental Health annual report, of 11,000 students who indicated sleep disturbances on intake, only 44 had that concern prioritized by clinicians.[107] College health communities could improve their practices by offering continuing education opportunities about sleep for college health providers.

In spring 2019, the National Collegiate Athletic Association (NCAA) issued its first consensus statement regarding sleep in collegiate varsity athletes,[108] and it is likely that more organizations will follow suit. The top recommendations included sleep screening and evidence-based education programs for both student-athletes and athletic staff members. When sleep questions are included as part of a universal behavioral health screening program, more than 10% of students request support for their sleep concerns.[109] Screening for disturbances in students' sleep in health services intake questionnaires, athlete preparticipation examinations, and as part of academic advising appointments could identify students with undiagnosed sleep disorders and those most in need of behavior sleep medicine.

Intervention Studies

Experimental studies of the impact of sleep education on sleep behaviors have ranged from studies of simple text messages and public media campaigns to intensive, semester-long courses on sleep.[8,110] Several before-after studies have shown that students report reduced sleep latency, fewer maladaptive beliefs about sleep, and a better understanding of sleep hygiene practices after receiving sleep education from an educational Web site with personalized feedback,[111] or a 3-hour in-person course.[112] Two months after taking a full-semester course on sleep, students showed better sleep hygiene and reduced sleep latency, as well as improved symptoms of depression and anxiety, compared with students taking another psychology class.[113]

A recent systematic review found that education about sleep hygiene was associated with modest effect sizes in improving student sleep, but cognitive behavior therapy for insomnia (CBTi) interventions were much more effective.[114] In college students, rumination and repetitive negative thinking mediate the relationship between stress and sleep quality,[90,115] and subjective stress explains more of the variance in students' PSQI scores than do sleep hygiene factors.[7] Low-cost digital delivery of CBTi improves both sleep and mental health outcomes in college students,[116] and an e-mail–delivered CBTi program outperformed a stress management module of similar length.[117]

SUMMARY

Sleep health emerges as an underused, highly requested, cost-efficient way to improve students' well-being and academic performance.[118] A research challenge for any examination of student success will be to sufficiently address multicollinearity among behavioral, social, and environmental variables that correlate with sleep. As university staff and administrators work toward reducing racial, ethnic, gender, and socioeconomic disparities in measures of academic success, they would be well served to prioritize Maslow's heirarchy of needs and Bloom's taxonomy.

DISCLOSURE

The author has nothing to disclose.

REFERENCES

1. Crowley SJ, Wolfson AR, Tarokh L, et al. An update on adolescent sleep: new evidence informing the perfect storm model. J Adolesc 2018;67:55–65.
2. Twenge JM, Krizan Z, Hisler G. Decreases in self-reported sleep duration among U.S. adolescents 2009-2015 and association with new media screen time. Sleep Med 2017;39:47–53.
3. School health policies and practices study. 2014. Available at: https://www.cdc.gov/healthyyouth/data/shpps/pdf/shpps-508-final_101315.pdf. Accessed June 29, 2019.
4. Park H, Chiang JJ, Irwin MR, et al. Developmental trends in sleep during adolescents' transition to young adulthood. Sleep Med 2019;60:202–10.
5. Badr MS, Belenky G, Bliwise DL, et al. Recommended amount of sleep for a healthy adult: a joint consensus statement of the American academy of sleep medicine and sleep research society. J Clin Sleep Med 2015;11(06):591–2.
6. American College Health Association National College Health. Assessment summary reports. Available at: https://www.acha.org/NCHA/ACHA-NCHA_Data/Publications_and_Reports/NCHA/Data/Reports_ACHA-NCHAIIc.aspx. Accessed June 1, 2019.
7. Lund HG, Reider BD, Whiting AB, et al. Sleep patterns and predictors of disturbed sleep in a large population of college students. J Adolesc Health 2010;46(2):124–32.
8. Orzech KM, Salafsky DB, Hamilton LA. The state of sleep among college students at a large public university. J Am Coll Health 2011;59(7):612–9.
9. Becker SP, Jarrett MA, Luebbe AM, et al. Sleep in a large, multi-university sample of college students: sleep problem prevalence, sex differences, and mental health correlates. Sleep Health 2018;4(2):174–81.
10. Hartmann ME, Prichard JR. Calculating the contribution of sleep problems to undergraduates' academic success. Sleep Health 2018;4(5):463–71.
11. Taylor DJ, Vatthauer KE, Bramoweth AD, et al. The role of sleep in predicting college academic performance: is it a unique predictor? Behav Sleep Med 2013;11(3):159–72.
12. Gomes AA, Tavares J, de Azevedo MH, et al. Sleep and academic performance in undergraduates: a multi-measure, multi-predictor approach. Chronobiol Int 2011;28(9):786–801.
13. Chen W, Chen J. Consequences of inadequate sleep during the college years: sleep deprivation, grade point average, and college graduation. Prev Med 2019;124:23–8.
14. Chen W, Chen J. Sleep deprivation and the development of leadership and need for cognition during the college years. J Adolesc 2019;73:95–9.
15. Peters BR, Joireman J, Ridgway RL. Individual differences in the consideration of future consequences scale correlate with sleep habits, sleep quality, and GPA in university students. Psychol Rep 2005;96(3):817–24.
16. Phillips AJK, Clerx WM, O'Brien CS, et al. Irregular sleep/wake patterns are associated with poorer academic performance and delayed circadian and sleep/wake timing. Sci Rep 2017;7(1):3216.
17. Okano K, Kaczmarzyk JR, Dave N, et al. Sleep quality, duration, and consistency are associated with better academic performance in college students. NPJ Sci Learn 2019;4:16.
18. Curcio G, Ferrara M, De Gennaro L. Sleep loss, learning capacity and academic performance. Sleep Med Rev 2006;10(5):323–37.
19. Huang S, Deshpande A, Yeo S, et al. Sleep restriction impairs vocabulary learning when adolescents cram for exams: the need for sleep study. Sleep 2016;39(9):1681–90.
20. Lo JC, Ong JL, Leong RLF, et al. Cognitive performance, sleepiness, and mood in partially sleep deprived adolescents: the need for sleep study. Sleep 2016;39(3):687–98.
21. Gao C, Terlizzese T, Scullin MK. Short sleep and late bedtimes are detrimental to educational learning and knowledge transfer: an investigation of individual differences in susceptibility. Chronobiol Int 2019;36(3):307–18.
22. Scullin MK. The eight hour sleep challenge during final exams week. Teach Psychol 2019;46(1):55–63.
23. Spoormaker VI, Verbeek I, van den Bout J, et al. Initial validation of the SLEEP-50 questionnaire. Behav Sleep Med 2005;3(4):227–46.
24. Gaultney JF. The prevalence of sleep disorders in college students: impact on academic performance. J Am Coll Health 2010;59(2):91–7.
25. Gaultney JF. Risk for sleep disorder measured during students' first college semester may predict institutional retention and grade point average over a 3-year period, with indirect effects through self-efficacy. J Coll Stud Ret 2016;18(3):333–59.
26. Khassawneh BY, Alkhatib LL, Ibnian AM, et al. The association of snoring and risk of obstructive sleep apnea with poor academic performance among university students. Sleep Breath 2018;22(3):831–6.

27. Norbury R, Evans S. Time to think: subjective sleep quality, trait anxiety and university start time. Psychiatry Res 2019;271:214–9.

28. Eliasson AH, Lettieri CJ, Eliasson AH. Early to bed, early to rise! sleep habits and academic performance in college students. Sleep Breath 2010; 14(1):71–5.

29. Nahmod NG, Lee S, Master L, et al. Later high school start times associated with longer actigraphic sleep duration in adolescents. Sleep 2019;42(2). https://doi.org/10.1093/sleep/zsy212.

30. Bowers JM, Moyer A. Effects of school start time on students' sleep duration, daytime sleepiness, and attendance: a meta-analysis. Sleep Health 2017; 3(6):423–31.

31. Carrell SE, Maghakian T, West JE. A's from zzzz's? the causal effect of school start time on the academic achievement of adolescents. Am Econ J Econ Policy 2011;3(3):62–81.

32. Irwin MR. Why sleep is important for health: a psychoneuroimmunology perspective. Annu Rev Psychol 2015;66:143–72.

33. Orzech KM, Acebo C, Seifer R, et al. Sleep patterns are associated with common illness in adolescents. J Sleep Res 2014;23(2):133–42.

34. Milewski MD, Skaggs DL, Bishop GA, et al. Chronic lack of sleep is associated with increased sports injuries in adolescent athletes. J Pediatr Orthop 2014;34(2):129.

35. Raikes AC, Athey A, Alfonso-Miller P, et al. Insomnia and daytime sleepiness: risk factors for sports-related concussion. Sleep Med 2019;58: 66–74.

36. Saylor J, Ji X, Calamaro CJ, et al. Does sleep duration, napping, and social jetlag predict hemoglobin A1c among college students with type 1 diabetes mellitus? Diabetes Res Clin Pract 2019; 148:102–9.

37. Wong ML, Lau EYY, Wan JHY, et al. The interplay between sleep and mood in predicting academic functioning, physical health and psychological health: a longitudinal study. J Psychosom Res 2013;74(4):271–7.

38. Hunter JC, Hayden KM. The association of sleep with neighborhood physical and social environment. Public Health 2018;162:126–34.

39. Robbins R, Jean-Louis G, Gallagher RA, et al. Examining social capital in relation to sleep duration, insomnia, and daytime sleepiness. Sleep Med 2019;60:165–72.

40. Sexton-Radek K, Hartley A. College residential sleep environment. Psychol Rep 2013;113(3): 903–7.

41. Peltz JS, Rogge RD. The indirect effects of sleep hygiene and environmental factors on depressive symptoms in college students. Sleep Health 2016;2(2):159–66.

42. Foulkes L, McMillan D, Gregory AM. A bad night's sleep on campus: an interview study of first-year university students with poor sleep quality. Sleep Health 2019;5(3):280–7.

43. Qin P, Brown CA. Sleep practices of university students living in residence. Int J High Edu 2017;6(5): 14–25.

44. LeBourgeois MK, Hale L, Chang A, et al. Digital media and sleep in childhood and adolescence. Pediatrics 2017;140(Suppl 2):S96.

45. Chinoy ED, Duffy JF, Czeisler CA. Unrestricted evening use of light-emitting tablet computers delays self-selected bedtime and disrupts circadian timing and alertness. Physiol Rep 2018;6(10): e13692.

46. Matar Boumosleh J, Jaalouk D. Depression, anxiety, and smartphone addiction in university students- A cross sectional study. PLoS One 2017; 12(8):e0182239.

47. You Z, Zhang Y, Zhang L, et al. How does self-esteem affect mobile phone addiction? the mediating role of social anxiety and interpersonal sensitivity. Psychiatry Res 2019;271:526–31.

48. Murdock KK, Horissian M, Crichlow-Ball C. Emerging adults' text message use and sleep characteristics: a multimethod, naturalistic study. Behav Sleep Med 2017;15(3):228–41.

49. Rosen L, Carrier LM, Miller A, et al. Sleeping with technology: cognitive, affective, and technology usage predictors of sleep problems among college students. Sleep Health 2016;2(1):49–56.

50. Duggan KA, McDevitt EA, Whitehurst LN, et al. To nap, perchance to DREAM: a factor analysis of college students' self-reported reasons for napping. Behav Sleep Med 2018;16(2):135–53.

51. Ye L, Hutton Johnson S, Keane K, et al. Napping in college students and its relationship with nighttime sleep. J Am Coll Health 2015;63(2):88–97.

52. Herrmann ML, Palmer AK, Sechrist MF, et al. College students' sleep habits and their perceptions regarding its effects on quality of life. International Journal of Studies in Nursing 2018;3(2):7.

53. Thompson K, Wood D, Davis MacNevin P. Sex differences in the impact of secondhand harm from alcohol on student mental health and university sense of belonging. Addict Behav 2019;89: 57–64.

54. McCabe SE, West BT, Teter CJ, et al. Trends in medical use, diversion, and nonmedical use of prescription medications among college students from 2003 to 2013: connecting the dots. Addict Behav 2014;39(7):1176–82.

55. Smith JM, Mader J, Szeto ACH, et al. Cannabis use for medicinal purposes among Canadian university students. Can J Psychiatry 2019;64(5):351–5.

56. Boehm MA, Lei QM, Lloyd RM, et al. Depression, anxiety, and tobacco use: overlapping

impediments to sleep in a national sample of college students. J Am Coll Health 2016;64(7): 565–74.

57. Kelly CK, Prichard JR. Demographics, health, and risk behaviors of young adults who drink energy drinks and coffee beverages. J Caffeine Res 2016;6(2):73–81.

58. Champlin SE, Pasch KE, Perry CL. Is the consumption of energy drinks associated with academic achievement among college students? J Prim Prev 2016;37(4):345–59.

59. Clegg-Kraynok MM, McBean AL, Montgomery-Downs HE. Sleep quality and characteristics of college students who use prescription psychostimulants nonmedically. Sleep Med 2011;12(6): 598–602.

60. Alamir YA, Zullig KJ, Wen S, et al. Association between nonmedical use of prescription drugs and sleep quality in a large college student sample. Behav Sleep Med 2019;17(4):470–80.

61. Goodhines PA, Gellis LA, Kim J, et al. Self-medication for sleep in college students: concurrent and prospective associations with sleep and alcohol behavior. Behav Sleep Med 2019;17(3):327–41.

62. Conroy DA, Kurth ME, Strong DR, et al. Marijuana use patterns and sleep among community-based young adults. J Addict Dis 2016;35(2):135–43.

63. Wong MM, Craun EA, Bravo AJ, et al. Insomnia symptoms, cannabis protective behavioral strategies, and hazardous cannabis use among U.S. college students. Exp Clin Psychopharmacol 2019. https://doi.org/10.1037/pha0000273.

64. Koob GF, Colrain IM. Alcohol use disorder and sleep disturbances: a feed-forward allostatic framework. Neuropsychopharmacology 2019. https://doi.org/10.1038/s41386-019-0446-0.

65. Caviness CM, Anderson BJ, Stein MD. Impact of nicotine and other stimulants on sleep in young adults. J Addict Med 2019;13(3):209–14.

66. Patel NP, Grandner MA, Xie D, et al. "Sleep disparity" in the population: poor sleep quality is strongly associated with poverty and ethnicity. BMC Public Health 2010;10(1):475.

67. Kalousová L, Xiao B, Burgard SA. Material hardship and sleep: Results from the Michigan recession and recovery study. Sleep Health 2019;5(2): 113–27.

68. Grandner MA, Hale L, Jackson N, et al. Perceived racial discrimination as an independent predictor of sleep disturbance and daytime fatigue. Behav Sleep Med 2012;10(4):235–49.

69. Chao RC, Mallinckrodt B, Wei M. Co-occurring presenting problems in African American college clients reporting racial discrimination distress. Prof Psychol Res Pract 2012;43(3):199–207.

70. John-Henderson NA, Palmer CA, Thomas A. Life stress, sense of belonging and sleep in american indian college students. Sleep Health 2019. https://doi.org/10.1016/j.sleh.2019.04.001.

71. Martinez MS, Grandner AM, Nazmi A, et al. Pathways from food insecurity to health outcomes among California university students. Nutrients 2019;11(6). https://doi.org/10.3390/nu11061419.

72. Teixeira L, Lowden A, da Luz AA, et al. Sleep patterns and sleepiness of working college students. Work 2012;41(Suppl 1):5550–2.

73. Barone TL. "Sleep is on the back burner": working students and sleep. Soc Sci J 2017;54(2): 159–67.

74. Thurston RC, Chang Y, Matthews KA, et al. Association of sexual harassment and sexual assault with midlife women's mental and physical health. JAMA Intern Med 2019;179(1):48–53.

75. Gallegos AM, Trabold N, Cerulli C, et al. Sleep and interpersonal violence: a systematic review. Trauma Violence Abuse 2019. https://doi.org/10.1177/1524838019852633. 1524838019852633.

76. Dai H, Ingram DG, Taylor JB. Hierarchical and mediation analysis of disparities in very short sleep among sexual minority youth in the U.S., 2015. Behav Sleep Med 2019;1–14. https://doi.org/10.1080/15402002.2019.1607738.

77. Jones SG, Benca RM. Circadian disruption in psychiatric disorders. Sleep Med Clin 2015;10(4): 481–93.

78. Rumble ME, White KH, Benca RM. Sleep disturbances in mood disorders. Psychiatr Clin North Am 2015;38(4):743–59.

79. Xiao H, Carney DM, Youn SJ, et al. Are we in crisis? national mental health and treatment trends in college counseling centers. Psychol Serv 2017;14(4):407–15.

80. Kalb LG, Stapp EK, Ballard ED, et al. Trends in psychiatric emergency department visits among youth and young adults in the US. Pediatrics 2019; 143(4):e20182192.

81. Patalay P, Gage SH. Changes in millennial adolescent mental health and health-related behaviours over 10 years: a population cohort comparison study. Int J Epidemiol 2019. https://doi.org/10.1093/ije/dyz006.

82. Baglioni C, Nanovska S, Regen W, et al. Sleep and mental disorders: a meta-analysis of polysomnographic research. Psychol Bull 2016;142(9): 969–90.

83. Lee S, Kim H, Lee K. Association between sleep duration and attention-deficit hyperactivity disorder: a systematic review and meta-analysis of observational studies☆. J Affect Disord 2019;256: 62–9.

84. Tsai M, Huang Y. Attention-deficit/hyperactivity disorder and sleep disorders in children. Med Clin North Am 2010;94(3):615–32.

85. Andorko ND, Mittal V, Thompson E, et al. The association between sleep dysfunction and

psychosis-like experiences among college students. Psychiatry Res 2017;248:6–12.

86. Dietch JR, Taylor DJ, Sethi K, et al. Psychometric evaluation of the PSQI in U.S. college students. J Clin Sleep Med 2016;12(8):1121–9.

87. Begdache L, Kianmehr H, Sabounchi N, et al. Principal component regression of academic performance, substance use and sleep quality in relation to risk of anxiety and depression in young adults. Trends Neurosci Edu 2019;15:29–37.

88. Berger AT, Wahlstrom KL, Widome R. Relationships between sleep duration and adolescent depression: a conceptual replication. Sleep Health 2019; 5(2):175–9.

89. Van Dyk TR, Thompson RW, Nelson TD. Daily bidirectional relationships between sleep and mental health symptoms in youth with emotional and behavioral problems. J Pediatr Psychol 2016; 41(9):983–92.

90. Li Y, Gu S, Wang Z, et al. Relationship between stressful life events and sleep quality: rumination as a mediator and resilience as a moderator. Front Psychiatry 2019;10:348.

91. Liu JCJ, Verhulst S, Massar SAA, et al. Sleep deprived and sweating it out: the effects of total sleep deprivation on skin conductance reactivity to psychosocial stress. Sleep 2015;38(1):155–9.

92. Schwarz J, Gerhardsson A, van Leeuwen W, et al. Does sleep deprivation increase the vulnerability to acute psychosocial stress in young and older adults? Psychoneuroendocrinology 2018;96: 155–65.

93. McMakin DL, Dahl RE, Buysse DJ, et al. The impact of experimental sleep restriction on affective functioning in social and nonsocial contexts among adolescents. J Child Psychol Psychiatry 2016;57(9):1027–37.

94. Blumenthal H, Taylor DJ, Cloutier RM, et al. The links between social anxiety disorder, insomnia symptoms, and alcohol use disorders: findings from a large sample of adolescents in the United States. Behav Ther 2019;50(1):50–9.

95. Ben Simon E, Walker MP. Sleep loss causes social withdrawal and loneliness. Nat Commun 2018;9(1): 1–9.

96. Liu J, Tu Y, Lai Y, et al. Associations between sleep disturbances and suicidal ideation, plans, and attempts in adolescents: a systematic review and meta-analysis. Sleep 2019;42(6). https://doi.org/10.1093/sleep/zsz054.

97. Littlewood DL, Kyle SD, Carter L-A, et al. Short sleep duration and poor sleep quality predict next-day suicidal ideation: an ecological momentary assessment study. Psychol Med 2018;49: 403–11.

98. Bernert RA, Hom MA, Iwata NG, et al. Objectively assessed sleep variability as an acute warning sign of suicidal ideation in a longitudinal evaluation of young adults at high suicide risk. J Clin Psychiatry 2017;78(6):e687.

99. Cairns KE, Yap MBH, Pilkington PD, et al. Risk and protective factors for depression that adolescents can modify: a systematic review and meta-analysis of longitudinal studies. J Affect Disord 2014;169:61–75.

100. Milojevich HM, Lukowski AF. Sleep and mental health in undergraduate students with generally healthy sleep habits. PLoS One 2016;11(6): e0156372.

101. Bei B, Ong JC, Rajaratnam SMW, et al. Chronotype and improved sleep efficiency independently predict depressive symptom reduction after group cognitive behavioral therapy for insomnia. J Clin Sleep Med 2015;11(9):1021–7.

102. Mason EC, Harvey AG. Insomnia before and after treatment for anxiety and depression. J Affect Disord 2014;168:415–21.

103. Counts CJ, Grubin FC, John-Henderson NA. Childhood socioeconomic status and risk in early family environments: predictors of global sleep quality in college students. Sleep Health 2018; 4(3):301–6.

104. Rojo-Wissar DM, Davidson RD, Beck CJ, et al. Sleep quality and perceived health in college undergraduates with adverse childhood experiences. Sleep Health 2019;5(2):187–92.

105. Mindell JA, Bartle A, Wahab NA, et al. Sleep education in medical school curriculum: a glimpse across countries. Sleep Med 2011;12(9):928–31.

106. Meltzer LJ, Phillips C, Mindell JA. Clinical psychology training in sleep and sleep disorders. J Clin Psychol 2009;65(3):305–18.

107. Center for collegiate mental health 2018 annual report. Available at: https://sites.psu.edu/ccmh/files/2019/01/2018-Annual-Report-1.30.19-ziytkb.pdf. Accessed June 29, 2019.

108. Kroshus E, Wagner J, Wyrick D, et al. Wake up call for collegiate athlete sleep: narrative review and consensus recommendations from the NCAA inter-association task force on sleep and wellness. Br J Sports Med 2019;53(12):731–6.

109. Shepardson RL, Funderburk JS. Implementation of universal behavioral health screening in a university health setting. J Clin Psychol Med Settings 2014;21(3):253–66.

110. Jones KE, Evans R, Forbes L, et al. Research on freshman and sleeping habits: a text message-based sleep intervention. J Am Coll Health 2019;1–8. https://doi.org/10.1080/07448481.2019.1626860.

111. Hershner S, O'Brien LM. Sleep education for college students. J Clin Sleep Med 2018;14(7):1271–2.

112. Kloss JD, Nash CO, Walsh CM, et al. A "Sleep 101" program for college students improves sleep

hygiene knowledge and reduces maladaptive beliefs about sleep. Behav Med 2016;42(1):48–56.

113. Baroni A, Bruzzese J, Di Bartolo CA, et al. Impact of a sleep course on sleep, mood and anxiety symptoms in college students: a pilot study. J Am Coll Health 2018;66(1):41–50.

114. Friedrich A, Schlarb AA. Let's talk about sleep: a systematic review of psychological interventions to improve sleep in college students. J Sleep Res 2018;27(1):4–22.

115. Amaral AP, Soares MJ, Pinto AM, et al. Sleep difficulties in college students: the role of stress, affect and cognitive processes. Psychiatry Res 2018;260: 331–7.

116. Freeman D, Sheaves B, Goodwin GM, et al. The effects of improving sleep on mental health (OASIS): a randomised controlled trial with mediation analysis. Lancet Psychiatry 2017;4(10): 749–58.

117. Trockel M, Manber R, Chang V, et al. An e-mail delivered CBT for sleep-health program for college students: effects on sleep quality and depression symptoms. J Clin Sleep Med 2011;7(3):276.

118. Prichard JR, Hartmann ME. Follow-up to Hartmann & Prichard: should universities invest in promoting healthy sleep? A question of academic and economic significance. Sleep Health 2019. https://doi.org/10.1016/j.sleh.2019.01.006.

Insomnia and Cognitive Performance

Janeese A. Brownlow, PhD[a,b,*], Katherine E. Miller, PhD[c], Philip R. Gehrman, PhD, CBSM[b,c]

KEYWORDS

- Insomnia • Attention • Memory • Concentration • Executive function

KEY POINTS

- Standardization in cognitive measures is warranted to strengthen the interpretability of insomnia findings.
- The use of normative data is recommended to further examine the clinical significance of cognitive impairments in insomnia.
- A detailed description of diagnostic procedures and measures for the classification of insomnia would increase the ability to generalize from study findings.

Insomnia is one of the most common subjective sleep complaints in the general and clinical adult populations,[1,2] and is characterized by persistent difficulty with the initiation and/or maintenance of sleep or nonrestorative sleep, with daytime functional impairment and distress among the core diagnostic features.[3] Prevalence estimates for insomnia symptoms range between 30% and 50%[4] in the general adult population and up to 80%[2] in patients with psychiatric illnesses. Although prevalence rates are high, only about 6% to 10% of adults have insomnia that meets full diagnostic criteria for insomnia disorder.[3,5,6] Daytime functional impairment is part of the diagnostic criteria for insomnia; however, the exact nature of the relation between insomnia and daytime cognitive impairments is not completely understood, and the few studies to investigate this relationship have produced inconsistent findings.

Collectively, the insomnia literature has primarily focused on cognitive domains of attention, memory, and executive function (**Table 1**), and to a lesser degree concentration. This article provides a succinct summary of these findings.

INSOMNIA AND COGNITIVE DOMAINS OF FUNCTIONING

Insomnia and Attention

Attention is the most extensively studied neurobehavioral domain in relation to insomnia. However, the findings are difficult to synthesize and understand because of the various attentional tasks that have been used (ie, focused, sustained, or shift).[2] Focused attention requires the selection of targeted information for additional processing, often at the expense of focusing on other stimuli.[7] Focused attention, known as simple attention, tasks require the patient to respond to a specific stimulus while ignoring the distractor stimuli. There have been some studies that reported significant group differences on focused attention tasks[8]; however, most of the studies examining focused attention in patients with insomnia compared with controls found no significant group differences.[9–12]

Sustained attention, known as vigilance, involves the capacity to maintain alertness or vigilance over a period of time.[7] Sustained attention

[a] Department of Psychology, College of Health & Behavioral Sciences, Delaware State University, 1200 North DuPont Highway, Dover, DE 19901, USA; [b] Department of Psychiatry, Perelman School of Medicine at the University of Pennsylvania, 3535 Market Street, Suite 670, Philadelphia, PA 19104, USA; [c] Mental Illness Research, Education, and Clinical Center, Corporal Michael J. Crescenz Veterans Affairs Medical Center, 3900 Woodland Avenue, Philadelphia, PA 19104, USA
* Corresponding author. Department of Psychology, College of Health & Behavioral Sciences, Delaware State University, 1200 North DuPont Highway, Dover, DE 19901.
E-mail address: jbrownlow@desu.edu

Sleep Med Clin 15 (2020) 71–76
https://doi.org/10.1016/j.jsmc.2019.10.002

Table 1
Neurocognitive domains and functions assessed in insomnia

Neurocognitive Domain	Cognitive Functions Assessed	Test/Dependent Variables
Attention	Focused	Simple vigilance test
		Simple alertness test
		Simple reaction time
		Continuous performance test
		Digit span (forward)
		Visual tracking
		Word detection
		Letter search
		Simple auditory reaction time
		Go/no-go task
	Sustained	Persistence of vigilance task
		Continuous performance test
		Vigilance detection test
		Wilkinson auditory vigilance test
		Visual vigilance
		Simple psychomotor vigilance task
		Complex psychomotor vigilance task
	Shifting	Switching attention task
		Complex reaction time
		Divided attention
		Wilkinson 4 choice reaction time
		Four choice serial reaction time test
Memory	Working	Digit span (backward)
		Letter number sequencing
		Memory and search task
		Addition (2 digit)
		2-Back memory task
	Implicit/explicit	Episodic memory
		Audioverbal learning test
		Hopkins verbal learning test
		Verbal paired associates
		Visual reproductions
		Word recognition
		Visual recognition
		Work memory test of free recall
		Procedural memory (consolidation)
		Declarative memory (consolidation)
Executive function	Cognitive flexibility	Trail making test B
	Inhibitory control	Controlled oral word association task
		Semantic memory
		Stroop test
		Wisconsin card sorting test
		Logical reasoning
		Proof reading
		Verbal fluency (phonemic)
		Verbal fluency (semantic)
		Go/no-go task
		Switching attention task
		Stop-signal task
		Color-word interference task

tasks place a greater demand on anticipatory readiness than focused attention, and the capacity of an individual to maintain attention declines over time.[2] In contrast with focused attention, the results are less conclusive for sustained attention. There is discordance regarding findings of speed and accuracy on sustained attention tasks in patients with insomnia versus controls. For instance, some studies report that patients with insomnia are less accurate and slower on sustained attention tasks,[13–15] whereas other studies have not shown this relationship.[9,15] Some of the discordance may be attributed to the type of vigilance tasks incorporated, particularly those including distractor stimuli.

The most complex attentional task is shifting attention, which requires the ability to be flexible and adaptable in order to modify the focus of attention.[7] Compared with focused and sustained attention, shifting attention requires a greater degree of cognitive involvement because of the responses requiring adaptations based on the stimulus presented.[2] The findings regarding shifting attention in patients with insomnia and good sleepers have been mixed. Some studies report significant group differences, with patients with insomnia reporting greater performance deficits than good sleepers,[11,16] whereas other studies found no significant group differences between patients with insomnia and controls.[17,18]

More recently, studies have investigated the functioning of attentional networks and vigilance in patients with insomnia. One study concluded that there were no significant group effects between patients with insomnia versus controls on tasks assessing alertness, orientation, and executive function.[19] In a systematic review examining sleep-related attentional bias, 6 of the 9 studies revealed statistically significant differences between patients with insomnia and controls, with medium to large effects.[20] Not surprisingly, these studies found that individuals with insomnia show a greater attentional bias toward sleep-related stimuli than good sleepers. However, the review concluded that the role of sleep-related attentional bias in the development and maintenance of insomnia needs further investigation.

Insomnia and Memory

Several studies have investigated group differences between patients with insomnia and good sleepers on memory tasks. The most commonly evaluated memory tasks in the insomnia literature are working memory, and implicit and explicit memory. Working memory tasks are active tasks requiring individuals to hold and manipulate information in their minds over brief intervals.[2] Implicit (procedural) memory tasks require individuals to learn new skills or abilities, whereas explicit (declarative) memory tasks require individuals to learn new material and recall the information after either a short or long delay.[21] Collectively, findings are mixed, with some studies reporting impaired memory performance in patients with insomnia compared with good sleepers,[4,16,22] whereas others reported no significant group differences.[8,9,14,23,24]

One study provided an explanation for the group differences in patients with insomnia versus controls on memory tasks, suggesting that patients with insomnia may have a susceptibility to declarative memory interference.[25] A recent meta-analytical review reported mild but not definitive working memory deficits in patients with insomnia compared with controls.[26] The review suggested several methodological concerns regarding the selected studies, including nonmatched demographic characteristics, level of expertise in the administration of the neurobehavioral tests, the comparability of findings among different studies, and the ability to generalize to subjects with acute versus chronic insomnia.[26]

Insomnia and Concentration

The insomnia literature has been limited in scope regarding concentration problems (or the inability to think clearly) in patients with insomnia compared with good sleepers. Difficulty concentrating is one of the most common daytime complaints reported by individuals with insomnia.[27] The inability to concentrate might indicate problems with sustained attention or shifting attention. Some studies suggest there are subjective daytime impairments related to concentration problems. For example, 1 study found decreased mental concentration related to work performance in patients with insomnia compared with controls.[28] Using a single item to assess for concentration, another study found that patients with insomnia had difficulty concentrating during the day compared with good sleepers.[29] One of the limitations regarding the insomnia literature and its relation to concentration problems is that most of the studies have reported on subjective complaints, and there is limited evidence regarding objective cognitive measures to assess for difficulties with concentration.

Insomnia and Executive Function

The neurobehavioral domain of executive functioning is an emerging area of focus in the insomnia literature and includes several cognitive processes (to include aspects of attention and memory). The literature suggests that executive function does not represent a single cognitive ability but several distinct cognitive components focused on 3 core functions: inhibition (eg, inhibitory control, selective attention), working memory (eg, manipulation of information related to execution of task), and cognitive flexibility (eg, ability to make an adaptation based on action or thought).[30] The domain of executive function is responsible for higher-order cognitive processes such as planning, reasoning, inhibitory control, cognitive flexibility, and multitasking.[2,30,31]

The insomnia literature has provided mixed findings with regard to the 3 cognitive components of executive function. For instance, some studies have reported significant group differences between patients with insomnia and controls on tasks measuring inhibitory control,[4,16,32] whereas most studies reported no significant group differences.[18,33,34] A similar pattern of mixed findings has been observed on tasks of executive function assessing working memory, with some studies showing significant group differences between patients with insomnia and controls,[24,35] and other studies indicating no group effects.[22,36] Executive function tasks assessing cognitive flexibility have been more consistent, with most findings reporting no significant group differences between patients with insomnia and controls.[31]

Summary of Findings

To date, there have been 2 meta-analyses and 1 review of the daytime cognitive impairments seen in patients with insomnia, primarily focusing on attention and working memory, and some aspects of executive function. The review concluded that the studies provided limited evidence for a single and consistent reported cognitive impairment among patients with insomnia versus good-sleeper controls.[2] However, the review provided some generalizations centered on attentional tasks with a high cognitive load and tasks of working memory, suggesting cognitive impairments in patients with insomnia compared with controls.[2] The first meta-analysis reported small to moderate effects in patients with insomnia for tasks assessing episodic memory, problem solving, manipulation in working memory, and retention in working memory.[21] Although there were significant group differences on some measures of memory, the meta-analysis also concluded that no significant group differences were found on several measures assessing attention and aspects of executive function (ie, verbal fluency, cognitive flexibility).[21] In addition, this meta-analytical review concluded that further research focused on ecologically valid measures and normative data is necessary to more definitively establish the clinical relevance of cognitive impairments in insomnia.

The second published meta-analysis reported cognitive deficits of small to moderate magnitude in patients with insomnia versus good sleepers in reaction times of inhibitory control and cognitive flexibility tasks; however, no group differences were found regarding accuracy rates.[31] Working memory impairments were also found among patients with insomnia compared with controls. In contrast with the meta-analysis, a recent review reported no significant group differences between patients with insomnia and controls on executive functioning tasks.[30] The review concluded that there were several methodological concerns relating to the variability of the methods used, the types of neurobehavioral tests that were administered, and the inconsistency in diagnostic criteria for primary insomnia across the various studies.[30]

Challenges with the Interpretation of Cognitive Findings in Insomnia

Several challenges and limitations have been proposed regarding the interpretation of cognitive findings in the insomnia literature. In general, the findings have been inconsistent regarding cognitive deficits in patients with insomnia compared with good sleeper controls. Many factors may account for the discrepancies between studies. Collectively, these challenges and limitations are focused on 3 key areas: methodology, definition of the insomnia group, and varying neurobehavioral tasks used to assess for cognitive function. First, methodological differences related to heterogeneity of the test population, small sample sizes, comparability of results across studies, and the ability to generalize to individuals with insomnia have all been issues with interpretation of findings.[21] Second, many of the studies have used qualitative and quantitative criteria to characterize patients with insomnia; however, the operational definitions significantly differ across studies, and the variation in selection criteria and assessment modalities used to confirm these criteria further limits insomnia findings.[2,21,31,37] Further, one issue that has not been raised is the timing of those individuals with acute versus chronic insomnia, and how the timeline of the disorder may affect cognitive performance. Third, several concerns focused on the administration and interpretation of cognitive measures have been noted. Specifically, regarding testing selection (eg, incompatibility/different classifications of cognitive tasks), testing protocols and conditions to include repeat testing and timing of tests have all been reported as barriers and potential confounds that could interfere with interpretation of study findings.[2] Standardization in cognitive measures is warranted to strengthen the interpretability of insomnia findings. Another plausible limitation is that many of the cognitive tasks used were developed and validated to assess for major deficits in individuals with traumatic brain injuries or neurologic disorders.[21] Therefore, the cognitive tasks used may not provide sufficient sensitivity to detect the subtle differences that are commonly reported in patients with insomnia.

SUMMARY

Insomnia is a major public health concern associated with daytime cognitive complaints. In general, the insomnia literature has been mixed regarding cognitive impairments in attention, memory, and executive function. Small to moderate effects have shown impairment on some attentional and working memory tasks in individuals with insomnia. However, these findings should be interpreted with care given the inconsistent methods used across studies.

DISCLOSURE

JAB's time was supported by a Center Grant from the National Institute of General Medical Sciences (Grant # 5P20GM103653-08). KEM's time was supported by Career Development Award Number IK2 CX001874 from the United States (U.S.) Department of Veterans Affairs Clinical Sciences R&D (CSRD) Service. The views expressed here are the authors' and do not necessarily represent the views of the Department of Veterans Affairs or the United States government.

REFERENCES

1. Roth T, Roehrs Insomnia T. Epidemiology, characteristics, and consequences. Clin Cornerstone 2003; 5(3):5–15.
2. Shekleton JA, Rogers NL, Rajaratnam SM. Searching for the daytime impairments of primary insomnia. Sleep Med Rev 2010;14:47–60.
3. American Psychiatric Association. Diagnostic and statistical manual of mental disorders, fifth edition (DSM5). Arlington (VA): American Psychiatric Association; 2013.
4. Fortier-Brochu E, Morin CM. Cognitive impairment in individuals with insomnia: clinical significance and correlates. Sleep 2014;37(11):1787–98.
5. Morin CM, Benca R. Chronic insomnia. Lancet 2012; 379:1129–41.
6. Buysse DJ. Insomnia. JAMA 2013;309:706–16.
7. Mirsky AF, Anthony BJ, Duncan CC, et al. Analysis of the elements of attention: a neuropsychological approach. Neuropsychol Rev 1991;2(2):109–45.
8. Vignola A, Lamoureux C, Bastien CH, et al. Effects of chronic insomnia and use of benzodiazepines on daytime performance in older adults. J Gerontol B Psychol Sci Soc Sci 2000;55(1):P54–62.
9. Orff HJ, Drummond SPA, Nowakowski S, et al. Discrepancy between subjective symptomatology and objective neuropsychological performance in insomnia. Sleep 2007;30(9):1205–11.
10. Edinger JD, Glenn DM, Bastien LA, et al. Slow wave sleep and waking cognitive performance II: findings among middle-aged adults with and without insomnia complaints. Physiol Behav 2000;70(1–2): 127–34.
11. Edinger JD, Means MK, Carney CE, et al. Psychomotor performance deficits and their relation to prior nights' sleep among individuals with primary insomnia. Sleep 2008;31(5):599–607.
12. Schneider C, Fulda S, Schulz H. Daytime variation in performance and tiredness/sleepiness ratings in patients with insomnia, narcolepsy, sleep apnea and normal controls. J Sleep Res 2004;13(4): 373–83.
13. Hauri PJ. Cognitive deficits in insomnia patients. Acta Neurol Belg 1997;97(2):113–7.
14. Varkevisser M, Kerkhof GA. Chronic insomnia and performance in a 24-h constant routine study. J Sleep Res 2005;14(1):49–59.
15. Altena E, Van Der Werf YD, Strijers RL, et al. Sleep loss affects vigilance: effects of chronic insomnia and sleep therapy. J Sleep Res 2008;17(3): 335–43.
16. Haimov I, Hanuka E, Horowitz Y. Chronic insomnia and cognitive functioning among older adults. Behav Sleep Med 2008;6(1):32–54.
17. Boyle J, Trick L, Johnsen S, et al. Next-day cognition, psychomotor function, and driving-related skills following nighttime administration of eszopiclone. Hum Psychopharmacol 2008;23(5):385–97.
18. Sagaspe P, Philip P, Schwartz S. Inhibitory motor control in apneic and insomniac patients: a stop task study. J Sleep Res 2007;16(4):381–7.
19. Perrier J, Chavoix C, Bocca ML. Functioning of the three attentional networks and vigilance in primary insomnia. Sleep Med 2015;16(12):1569–75.
20. Harris K, Spiegelhalder K, Espie CA, et al. Sleep-related attentional bias in insomnia: a state-of-the-science review. Clin Psychol Rev 2015;42:16–27.
21. Fortier-Brochu E, Beaulieu-Bonneau S, Ivers H, et al. Insomnia and daytime cognitive performance: a meta-analysis. Sleep Med Rev 2012;16(1):83–94.
22. Skekleton JA, Flynn-Evans EE, Miller B, et al. Neurobehavioral performance impairment in insomnia: relationships with self-reported sleep and daytime functioning. Sleep 2014;37(1):107–16.
23. Lovato N, Lack L, Wright H, et al. Working memory performance of older adults with insomnia. J Sleep Res 2013;22(3):251–7.
24. Cellini N, de Zambotti M, Covassin N, et al. Working memory impairment and cardiovascular hyperarousal in young primary insomniacs. Psychophysiology 2014;51(2):206–14.

25. Griessenberger H, Heib DP, Lechinger J, et al. Susceptibility to Declarative memory interference is pronounced in primary insomnia. PLoS One 2013;8(2): e57394.

26. Monteiro B, Candida M, Monteiro S, et al. Working memory dysfunction in insomniac adults: a systematic metanalytical review. Med Express 2016;3(2): M160302.

27. Roth T, Ancoli-Israel S. Daytime consequences and correlates of insomnia in the United States: results of the 1991 National Sleep Foundation Survey. II. Sleep 1999;22(Suppl 2):S354–8.

28. Leger D, Guilleminault C, Bader G, et al. Medical and socio-professional impact of insomnia. Sleep 2002;25(6):625–9.

29. Alapin I, Fichten CS, Libman E, et al. How is good and poor sleep in older adults and college students related to daytime sleepiness, fatigue, and ability to concentrate? J Psychosom Res 2000;49(5):381–90.

30. Ferreira ODL, deAlmondes KM. The executive functions in primary insomniacs: literature review. Perspectivas En Psicologia 2014;11(2):1–9.

31. Ballesio A, Aquino MRJV, Kyle SD, et al. Executive functions in insomnia disorder: a systematic review and exploratory meta-Analysis. Front Psychol 2019; 10:101.

32. Liu H, Wang D, Li Y, et al. Examination of daytime sleepiness and cognitive performance testing in patients with primary insomnia. PLoS One 2014;9(6): e100965.

33. Covassin N, de Zambotti M, Sarlo M, et al. Cognitive performance and cardiovascular markers of hyperarousal in primary insomnia. Int J Psychophysiol 2011;80(1):79–86.

34. Sivertsen B, Hysing M, Wehling E, et al. Neuropsychological performance in older insomniacs. Neuropsychol Dev Cogn B Aging Neuropsychol Cogn 2013;20(1):34–48.

35. Chen GH, Xia L, Wang F, et al. Patients with chronic insomnia have selective impairments in memory that are modulated by cortisol. Psychophysiology 2016; 53(10):1567–76.

36. Khassawneh BY, Bathgate CJ, Tsai SC, et al. Neurocognitive performance in insomnia disorder: the impact of hyperarousal and short sleep duration. J Sleep Res 2018;27(6):e12747.

37. Buysse DJ, Ancoli-Israel S, Edinger JD, et al. Recommendations for a standard research assessment of insomnia. Sleep 2006;29(9):1155–73.

Effect of Obstructive Sleep Apnea on Neurocognitive Performance

Gilbert Seda, MD, PhD*, Tony S. Han, MD

KEYWORDS

- Obstructive sleep apnea • Neurocognitive performance • Attention • Psychomotor function
- Learning • Memory • Executive functioning • Continuous positive airway pressure (CPAP)

KEY POINTS

- Obstructive sleep apnea can affect multiple cognitive domains with the most profound effects on mood, daytime sleepiness, and attention/vigilance. There are moderate effects on learning, memory, and executive functioning.
- Mechanisms of cognitive impairment in obstructive sleep apnea include intermittent hypoxemia, sleep deprivation and fragmentation, disruption of the hypothalamic-pituitary-adrenal-axis, and hypercapnia.
- Continuous positive airway pressure can ameliorate some of the cognitive deficits associated with obstructive sleep apnea but more data are needed to determine the effectiveness of other therapies.

INTRODUCTION

Obstructive sleep apnea (OSA) is a sleep disorder of the upper airway leading to recurrent oxyhemoglobin desaturations, sleep fragmentation, increased sympathetic autonomic activity, and intrathoracic pressure fluctuations during sleep. It is a common condition and the prevalence of OSA seems to be on the rise with 2% to 4% reported previously in 1993[1,2] and around 15% reported more recently.[3,4] Furthermore, most patients with OSA remain undiagnosed and untreated. There is a preponderance of evidence that moderate-to-severe OSA is an independent risk factor for hypertension in middle-aged adults as well as excessive daytime sleepiness (EDS).[5,6] OSA is also associated with other serious medical conditions, such as stroke, myocardial infarction, endocrine dysfunction, and depression.[7–9]

There has been growing interest in understanding the impact of OSA and sleep loss on neurocognitive performance. The need for sleep is conserved in all animal species. Yet, despite the ubiquity of sleep, the role of sleep in brain function is mostly a mystery. β-Amyloid protein has been implicated in the pathology of Alzheimer dementia. An animal model study in 2013 demonstrated increased clearance rate of β-amyloid protein during sleep, suggesting that sleep is a restorative process for the brain.[10] Improved cognition is often touted as a benefit of continuous positive airway pressure (CPAP) therapy for OSA. Although CPAP has been demonstrated to improve EDS and nocturnal blood pressure, the neurocognitive benefits are less clear.[11] In this article, the effect of OSA on cognitive performance is discussed. Possible mechanisms of action and effects of CPAP treatment are also be covered.

Pulmonary Medicine Department, Naval Medical Center San Diego, 34800 Bob Wilson Drive, San Diego, CA 92134, USA
* Corresponding author.
E-mail address: gilbert.seda@gmail.com

Sleep Med Clin 15 (2020) 77–85
https://doi.org/10.1016/j.jsmc.2019.10.001
1556-407X/20/Published by Elsevier Inc.

sleep.theclinics.com

NEUROCOGNITIVE FUNCTION

Brain function can be divided into several neurocognitive domains that are affected differentially by OSA and sleep loss (**Table 1**). Psychomotor function, attention, and vigilance have strong correlations with sleep loss. Learning and memory seem to be dependent on sleep quality and duration. Alterations in mood regulation may have implications for the development of depression and anxiety. Executive function involves the use of memory for planning, reasoning, and problem solving.

Attention and Vigilance

Vigilance is the ability to focus on a specific task over an extended period of time and is crucial for occupational tasks such as motor vehicle operation or industrial equipment monitoring. EDS is inversely correlated with vigilance and is a common feature of OSA, yet not all patients with OSA display EDS. In the Sleep Heart Health Study cohort of 6440 participants, only 46% with moderate-to-severe OSA reported an Epworth Sleepiness Score >10.[12] In addition, EDS as measured by psychomotor vigilance testing (PVT) and mean sleep latency testing does not seem to correlate with the severity of OSA.[13]

Excessive sleepiness due to OSA is a well-recognized cause of motor vehicle crashes, and there have been regulatory efforts to mitigate this risk, especially in commercial motor vehicle operators. The relative risk of motor vehicle crashes seems to be around 2 in patients with OSA based on retrospective data; however, OSA severity does not predict risk.[14–16] Risk of injury is also increased about 2-fold in patients with OSA involved in collisions.[15] CPAP treatment seems to reduce this risk significantly with a significant effect seen with at least 4 hours of nightly use.[15] Yet, there are clearly other significant contributing factors, such as subjective sleepiness and short habitual sleep duration. Short sleep duration has been shown to be a significant risk factor in a recent study that calculated the population-attributable fraction of crashes due to OSA to be 10% compared with 9% due to sleep duration less than 7 hours.[17] Other individual factors may be important in driving performance and vigilance. Twenty-three out of 38 patients with OSA had no significant decline in simulated driving performance despite short sleep duration less than 4 hours or exposure to ethanol in a study looking at resiliency of drivers.[18] The presence of OSA is a strong predictor of impaired vigilance and motor vehicle crashes yet there does not seem to be a correlation with OSA severity. Other factors, such as sleep duration and subjective sleepiness seem to be just as important.

Learning and Memory

Learning and memory are closely related and can be divided into verbal, visual, and procedural domains. Effective learning requires information processing, consolidation, and retrieval. There have been some studies attempting to assess the

Table 1
Effect of obstructive sleep apnea on cognitive domains

Cognitive Domain	Definition	Assessments	OSA Effect
Excessive daytime sleepiness	Urge to fall asleep	Epworth sleepiness score Mean sleep latency test	High
Attention and vigilance	Sustained focus while filtering out distractions	Psychomotor vigilance task Driving simulators	High
Learning and memory	Immediate and delayed recall of images, words, and procedures	Sustained working memory test Spatial span Logical memory test California Verbal Learning Test	Moderate
Psychomotor function	Manual coordination and dexterity	Mirror tracing task Sequential finger tapping task	Low
Executive function	Reasoning, planning, and problem solving	Stroop test Paced Auditory Serial Addition Test	Moderate

impact of OSA on different domains of memory and learning. A 2006 study by Naegele and colleagues[19] used an extensive battery of tests to discover mild memory deficits in patients with OSA compared with matched controls. There was also the finding of more rapid improvement in procedural tasks seen in controls. Deficits did not correlate with OSA severity but there was a relationship with educational level. A 2010 study comparing 60 patients with OSA with 60 healthy volunteers showed that patients with OSA had difficulty assimilating new information but did not have more difficulty retaining learned information, suggesting an effect on information consolidation.[20] These patients with OSA performed worse on verbal memory tests yet visual memory and attention were the same as controls.

A comprehensive review in 2003 by Beebe and colleagues[21] found that vigilance was markedly affected by OSA in all studies to that point. OSA also affected executive function substantially, but the effects on memory, intelligence, and visual and motor function were inconsistent, especially when compared with possibly outdated normative values. A more recent 2013 meta-analysis of 1413 participants with OSA and 1346 healthy controls found that OSA was associated with impaired verbal recall.[22] Both immediate and delayed verbal recall were impaired with moderate effect size compared with both controls and normative values. Visual memory was again not found to be affected by OSA and there was no correlation with OSA severity as defined by the apnea-hypopnea index (AHI).

Hoth and colleagues[23] attempted to separate the effects of hypoxemia and sleep disruption on cognitive function by studying 2 groups matched by age, sex, and AHI, but differed on severity of hypoxemia. The groups differed significantly on verbal memory, specifically verbal immediate recall tests with a large effect size. The surprising finding was that the group with more severe hypoxemia performed better on memory and learning tasks than the mild hypoxemia group. This finding suggests that intermittent hypoxemia may confer some type of adaptive advantage for memory and learning. This is in contrast to other studies which indicate that intermittent hypoxemia disrupts short and long-term memory.[24]

Psychomotor Function and Procedural Memory

Psychomotor tests are tests that assess the subject's ability to perceive instructions and perform motor responses often including the measurement of the speed of the reaction.[25]

Psychomotor function includes fine motor coordination, dexterity, and processing speed. Assessments of this domain include the mirror tracing task (MTT), the sequential finger tapping task (SFTT), and the motor sequence learning task (MST). One of the first studies on psychomotor function in OSA showed no psychomotor deficits in 28 patients with OSA compared with controls on MTT.[26] A review from 2004 concluded that, although vigilance was degraded by OSA with improvement after treatment, the impact on other domains such as psychomotor function was equivocal.[27] A more recent 2012 meta-review by Bucks and colleagues[28] showed no consistent effect of OSA on psychomotor function or language ability.

OSA does not seem to have much effect on baseline psychomotor performance, yet sleep-related consolidation of memory and learning seems to be impaired in OSA. A study by Landry and colleagues[29] compared SFTT performance in 12 patients with OSA with 12 controls during presleep training and after overnight sleep consolidation. There was no difference during presleep training; however, the control group showed greater improvement of 15.35% after sleep, compared with the OSA group, which showed only a 1.78% improvement. Sixteen patients with mild OSA underwent PVT and MST before and after overnight sleep in a 2012 study by Djonlagic and colleagues.[30] Controls had significantly more improvement in performance (14.7%) after overnight sleep than patients with mild OSA (1.1%). Performance correlated with arousal index but not with oxygen parameters. These findings are consistent with the hypothesis that OSA impairs procedural learning that occurs during sleep. The overall effect of OSA on memory seems to be focused on verbal domains. Procedural learning and executive function seem to be impaired in OSA.

Emotional Modulation

There seems to be a bidirectional relationship between the brain circuitry involved in sleep and emotional regulation. There are several studies that suggest an association between disrupted sleep and psychiatric disorders. Sleep deprivation and disruptions in rapid eye movement (REM) sleep are associated with mood disturbances.[31] One potential consequence of OSA is a decreased ability to self-regulate emotions. Beebe and Gozal[32] propose a prefrontal model of OSA. They hypothesize that OSA results in sleep disruption and intermittent hypoxemia and hypercapnia that impairs the restorative function of sleep and disrupts nocturnal cellular and chemical homeostasis. The result is OSA-associated prefrontal cortical dysfunction, which is manifest in behavioral, cognitive, and emotional dysfunction. Lee and colleagues[33] studied the association of depression in REM-related sleep-disordered breathing (SDB) using the Beck Depression Inventory (BDI) and Medical Outcomes Study Short-Form Health Survey (SF-36). REM-related SDB was associated with depressive symptoms in men but now women.

There are multiple studies that show an association of mood disorders with OSA. BaHammam and colleagues[34] reviewed the link between comorbid depression and OSA. Their review of cross-sectional studies demonstrated a higher prevalence of depression among patients with OSA in community and in sleep clinic samples. Similar findings were found by Garbarino and colleagues,[35] who conducted a systemic review and meta-analysis on the association of depression and anxiety in OSA. They reviewed 5 databases and found 73 articles investigating the association with OSA and depression and anxiety. The pooled prevalence of depression and anxiety symptoms in patients with OSA was reported to be 35%. Similarly, Acker and colleagues[36] conducted a study to determine the prevalence of depression in patients with OSA. The surveyed 447 patients, of whom 322 had an AHI greater than 9. Depression was assessed using the BDI-II with a score $\geq$14 and the World Health Organization WHO-5 Well-Being Index $\leq$13. Clinical depression was diagnosed in 21% of the sample. Furthermore, the severity of the OSA does not directly correlate with the severity of mood symptoms. Lee and colleagues[37] using the BDI and State-Trait Anxiety Inventory investigated anxiety and depression in association with OSA severity. Interestingly, anxiety and depressive symptoms were more prevalent in patients with mild OSA than those with severe OSA.

Executive Function

Executive function involves complex behaviors such as manipulating and processing information, successful planning and execution of plans, sustained concentration, good judgment and decision making, maintaining motivation, and emotional flexibility.[38] Borges and colleagues[39] evaluated executive function in 22 healthy adults with moderate-to-severe OSA compared with healthy controls with similar demographics using a test battery with 6 distinct cognitive domains. They found that the AHI did not correlate with executive

performance but mean oxygen saturation correlated with measurements of executive shifting and retrieval of long-term memory. In contrast, Olaithe and Bucks[40] conducted a meta-analysis of OSA and executive dysfunction before and after treatment. The reviewed 5 domains of executive function: shifting, updating, inhibition, generativity, and fluid reasoning. Their meta-analysis included 21 studies that examined OSA and executive functioning compared with controls and 19 studies that conducted the comparison before and after OSA treatment. They found that all 5 domains of executive function demonstrated medium to large impairments in patients with OSA independent of age and disease severity.

Several studies suggest impaired executive function associated with OSA. Idiaquez and colleagues[41] investigated whether cognitive impairment in OSA is related to autonomic alterations or nocturnal oxygen desaturation. Executive cognitive function was assessed using the Syndrom-Kurz, Trail Making Test B, and the Frontal Assessment Battery tests. They found that patients with OSA had autonomic alterations and impairment of executive cognitive function and that these variables were independently correlated with nocturnal hypoxemia. Executive cognitive function was not associated with autonomic alterations but it was associated with hypoxemia. Werli and colleagues[42] evaluated the effects of residual daytime sleepiness after appropriate treatment of OSA. They compared patients with OSA with and without daytime sleepiness. Cognitive function was assessed using a battery of tests to include the Wisconsin Card Sorting Test, Digit Span, Stroop Color-Word Test, Trail Making Tests A and B, Rey Auditory Verbal Learning Test, Verbal Fluency and Categories (FAS Test), and Codes. They found that patients with OSA and residual daytime sleepiness had impairment of executive function but no impairments in other cognitive domains. Yilmaz and colleagues[43] also investigated executive function in 28 newly diagnosed patients with OSA. They found EDS to be the most influential factor associated with impaired executive function.

Another potential mechanism for impaired executive function in patients with OSA is impaired slow-wave activity (SWA), a subtle measure of sleep disruption, daytime sleepiness, and impaired sleep regulation. Weichard and colleagues[44] examined the relationship between OSA and impaired dissipation of SWA. Children with improvement in SWA dissipation had improved attention and reduced externalizing behaviors. Christiansz and colleagues[45] studied SWA and executive function. They too found that SWA in children with OSA was associated with deficits in problem solving and efficiency during sustained attention.

MECHANISMS OF NEUROCOGNITIVE IMPAIRMENT

There are several possible mechanisms for neurocognitive impairment in patients with OSA. Nocturnal hypoxemia, hypercapnia, sleep deprivation, and sleep fragmentation can disrupt the neurochemical and cerebral blood flow during sleep. OSA may also disrupt the hypothalamic-pituitary-adrenal (HPA) axis resulting in alterations of cortisol activity.

Intermittent Hypoxemia

Daytime and nocturnal hypoxemia can disrupt cognitive functioning by altering the biochemical and hemodynamic state of the central nervous system.[46] Findley and colleagues[47] investigated cognitive impairment in patients with OSA and hypoxemia in comparison with patients with OSA without hypoxemia. Patients with OSA with hypoxemia had mean performance scores in the impaired range on measures of attention, concentration, complex problem solving, and short-term recall of verbal and spatial information. In contrast, the patients who had sleep apnea without hypoxemia had no mean performance scores in the impaired range. In a sample of elderly people, Blackwell and colleagues[48] conducted a population-based longitudinal study to investigate the association of OSA-associated nocturnal hypoxemia and cognitive decline over 3.4 to 5 years. Cognitive decline was assessed using the Modified Mini-Mental State Examination and the Trail Making Test B at baseline and 2 follow-up points. Nocturnal hypoxemia was related to a greater decline in the Modified Mini-Mental State Examination. For each 5-point increase in the oxygen desaturation index (oxygen desaturation index [ODI] = number of oxygen desaturations of $\geq 3\%$ per hour of sleep) there was an average annual decline of 0.36 points ($P = .01$).

There is also increasing data that OSA-associated cyclical intermittent hypoxemia may disrupt the blood-brain barrier (BBB), which maintains homeostasis in the central nervous system. Furthermore, the disruption of the BBB leads to changes in synaptic plasticity and disrupts the brains microenvironment leading to cognitive impairment.[49] Kim and colleagues[24] demonstrated that mice with 14 days of intermittent hypoxemia mimicking OSA disrupted the BBB resulting in hypomyelination and short- and long-term memory impairment.

Sleep Deprivation and Fragmentation

Sleep deprivation and fragmentation are also associated with impaired cognitive performance. Ward and colleagues[50] assessed the effects of 24 hours of sleep fragmentation or intermittent hypoxemia in a rat model of OSA. They found that sleep fragmentation impaired retention with spatial memory being the cognitive function being most susceptible. Pilcher and Huffcutt[51] conducted a meta-analysis on the effects of sleep deprivation on performance. They identified 19 studies with a total sample size of 1932. They concluded that sleep deprivation has the most profound effect on mood compared with cognitive and motor performance. Moreover, they found that partial sleep deprivation has a greater effect on functioning than long- or short-term sleep deprivation. Lim and Dinges[52] conducted a meta-analysis on the impact of short-term sleep deprivation on cognition. They reviewed 70 studies with 147 cognitive tests, which included 6 cognitive categories: simple attention, complex attention, working memory, processing speed, short-term memory, and reasoning. They found that short-term sleep deprivation has significant detrimental effects across most cognitive domains, with the largest effects on simple, sustained attention. Furthermore, tests of executive function and working memory are also robustly affected by even 1 night of sleep deprivation.

Hypercapnia

Although not all patients with OSA have daytime or nocturnal hypercapnia. Kung and colleagues[53] conducted a prospective case-controlled study evaluating the effects of hypercapnia on cognitive performance and memory function. They enrolled 39 obese patients with OSA and collected the arterial blood samples. Subjects completed the Pittsburgh sleep quality index, the Epworth Sleepiness Scale, and 6 cognitive tasks (the psychomotor vigilance task, the Stroup task, the Erickson flanker tasks, processing speed, verbal memory, and visual memory). Hypercapnic obese patients with OSA had lower scores with respect to processing speed and logical memory tests. The authors believe that hypercapnia and delayed reaction time and cognitive function tests and was correlated with deficits and logical memory but not verbal memory. A limitation of the study was that carbon dioxide levels were not measured during the neurocognitive tests.

Neuroendocrine Dysfunction

Previous studies associating OSA and HPA axis dysfunction are mixed. In a systemic review by Tomfohr and colleagues,[54] altered cortisol levels were not consistently related to OSA. This may be because of the confounding effect of obesity, infrequent sampling of cortisol, and studies having only one-time measurements of cortisol. Kritikou and colleagues[55] examined the relationship between OSA and the HPA axis and the effects of CPAP in 72 men and women. They found that OSA in nonobese men and slightly obese women is associated with HPA axis activation, similar, albeit stronger, compared with obese individuals with OSA. Furthermore, short-term CPAP use decreased cortisol levels compared with baseline, indicating that CPAP may have a protective effect against chronic activation of the HPA axis. Edwards and colleagues[56] investigated whether impaired cortisol explains the neurocognitive effects of OSA. They assessed 55 subjects with OSA over a 2-day period collecting cortisol levels every 2 hours. They found that OSA severity was associated with 24-hour cortisol levels. The AHI, ODI, and nighttime cortisol levels were associated with impaired learning, memory, and working memory.

TREATMENT OF OBSTRUCTIVE SLEEP APNEA AND NEUROCOGNITIVE PERFORMANCE

The Apnea Positive Pressure Long-term Efficacy Study was a 6-month randomized, double-blind, 2-arm, sham-controlled, multicenter trial to determine the neurocognitive effects of CPAP therapy on patients with OSA.[57] The study investigated 3 neurocognitive domains: attention and psychomotor function were measured using the Pathfinder Number Test-Total Time, learning and memory were assessed using the Buschke Selective Reminding Test-Sum Recall, and executive and frontal lobe function were assessed using the Sustained Working Memory Test-Overall Midday Score. There was only a significant difference in the executive and frontal lobe function testing at the 2-month CPAP visit but no difference at the 6-month visit. Furthermore, there was no difference with respect to attention and psychomotor function for learning and memory at the 2 6-month visits. The investigators interpret their findings by stating there is a complex OSA-neurocognitive relationship and that patients may use preexisting cognitive processes or enlisting compensatory processes before cognitive performances are detrimentally affected.

There are studies that suggest improvements in cognitive function with use of CPAP. Antic and colleagues[58] studied the role of CPAP adherence on neurocognitive function in patients with moderate-to-severe OSA. Neurocognitive function was assessed using the Brain Resource Company IntegNeuro test. Neurocognitive domains evaluated include verbal recall, choice reaction time, executive maze errors, and time to completion of the executive maze. Pre-CPAP and post-CPAP treatment results were compared, as were comparisons with a control group that did not use CPAP. The CPAP adherence group had improvements in verbal memory and executive function after 3 months; however, vigilance was not significantly improved with CPAP use. Richards and colleagues[59] conducted a quasi-experimental pilot clinical trial on 25 older adults with mild cognitive impairment and OSA to determine whether CPAP adherence had an effect on cognitive decline compared with similar patients who were nonadherent to CPAP. CPAP adherence was defined as CPAP use 4 or more hours per night over 1 year. The primary cognitive outcome was memory using the Hopkins Verbal Learning Test-Revised, and secondary measures included the digit symbol subtest from the West-Schuyler's Adult Intelligence Scale substitution test. The mild cognitive impairment and CPAP adherence group had significant improvements in psychomotor and cognitive processing speed at 1 year.

Other therapies for OSA may improve cognitive performance. Gupta and colleagues[60] conducted a prospective single-arm study to evaluate the long-term effects of an oral appliance on cardiovascular fitness and psychomotor performance in 30 patients with mild to moderate OSA. Psychomotor performance was assessed using the psychomotor vigilance test at time 0, 6 months, 1-year, and 2-year follow-ups. At 6 months, 1 year, and 2 years average response time and count of lapses improved with the oral appliance. Yu and colleagues[61] conducted a meta-analysis on neuropsychological functioning after adenotonsillectomy (AT). After 6 to 12 months of observation, they found significant improvements in attention-executive function and verbal ability in children with OSA treated with AT compared with their baseline level. Moreover, there was restoration of attention-executive function and memory in children with OSA after AT in comparison with healthy controls.

An area that requires further investigation is the neurocognitive effects of hypoglossal nerve stimulators for treatment of OSA. A 5-year outcome study evaluating the effectiveness of hypoglossal nerve stimulation showed that the treatment has long-term benefits for patients with moderate-to-severe OSA. Patient's had improvement in daytime sleepiness, quality of life, and decreased AHI.[62]

SUMMARY

OSA can affect several domains of neurocognitive performance to include attention and vigilance, memory and learning, psychomotor function, emotional regulation, and executive function. Proposed mechanisms include intermittent hypoxemia, sleep deprivation and fragmentation, hypercapnia, and disruption of the HPA axis. Continuous positive airway pressure can improve cognitive defects associated with OSA. More data are needed to determine whether other therapies improve cognitive function.

DISCLOSURE

The views expressed in this article are those of the authors and do not necessarily reflect the official policy or position of the Department of the Navy, Department of Defense, nor the U.S. Government.

REFERENCES

1. Young T, Palta M, Dempsey J, et al. The occurrence of sleep-disordered breathing among middle-aged adults. N Engl J Med 1993;328(17):1230–5.
2. Young T, Peppard PE, Gottlieb DJ. Epidemiology of obstructive sleep apnea: a population health perspective. Am J Respir Crit Care Med 2002; 165(9):1217–39.
3. Nakayama-Ashida Y, Takegami M, Chin K, et al. Sleep-disordered breathing in the usual lifestyle setting as detected with home monitoring in a population of working men in Japan. Sleep 2008;31: 419–25.
4. Franklin KA, Sahlin C, Stenlund H, et al. Sleep apnoea is a common occurrence in females. Eur Respir J 2013;41:610–5.
5. Peppard PE, Young T, Palta M, et al. Prospective study of the association between sleep-disordered breathing and hypertension. N Engl J Med 2000; 342(19):1378–84.
6. Marin JM, Agusti A, Villar I, et al. Association between treated and untreated obstructive sleep apnea and risk of hypertension. JAMA 2012;307: 2169–76.
7. Arzt M, Young T, Finn L, et al. Association of sleep-disordered breathing and the occurrence of stroke. Am J Respir Crit Care Med 2005;172(11): 1447–51.
8. Peppard PE, Szklo-Coxe M, Hla KM, et al. Longitudinal association of sleep-related breathing disorder and depression. Arch Intern Med 2006;166(16): 1709–15.
9. Aronsohn RS, Whitmore H, Van Cauter E, et al. Impact of untreated obstructive sleep apnea on glucose control in type 2 diabetes. Am J Respir Crit Care Med 2010;181(5):507–13.
10. Xie L, Kang H, Xu Q, et al. Sleep drives metabolite clearance from the adult brain. Science 2013; 342(6156):373–7.
11. Marin JM, Carrizo SJ, Vicente E, et al. Long-term cardiovascular outcomes in men with obstructive sleep apnoea-hypopnoea with or without treatment with continuous positive airway pressure: an observational study. Lancet 2005;365(9464): 1046–53.
12. Kapur VK, Baldwin CM, Resnick HE, et al. Sleepiness in patients with moderate to severe sleep-disordered breathing. Sleep 2005;28:472–7.
13. Sauter C, Asenbaum S, Popovic R, et al. Excessive daytime sleepiness in patients suffering from different levels of obstructive sleep apnoea syndrome. J Sleep Res 2000;9:293–301.
14. Tregear S, Reston J, Schoelles K, et al. Obstructive sleep apnea and risk of motor vehicle crash: systematic review and meta-analysis. J Clin Sleep Med 2009;5:573–81.
15. Karimi M, Hedner J, Häbel H, et al. Sleep apnea related risk of motor vehicle accidents is reduced by continuous positive airway pressure: Swedish Traffic Accident Registry data. Sleep 2015;38(3):341–9.
16. Tregear S, Reston J, Schoelles K, et al. Continuous positive airway pressure reduces risk of motor vehicle crash among drivers with obstructive sleep apnea: systematic review and meta-analysis. Sleep 2010;33(10):1373–80.
17. Gottlieb DJ, Ellenbogen JM, Bianchi MT, et al. Sleep deficiency and motor vehicle crash risk in the general population: a prospective cohort study. BMC Med 2018;16(1):44.
18. Vakulin A, Catcheside PG, Baulk SD, et al. Individual variability and predictors of driving simulator impairment in patients with obstructive sleep apnea. J Clin Sleep Med 2014;10(6):647–55.
19. Naegele B, Launois SH, Mazza S, et al. Which memory processes are affected in patients with obstructive sleep apnea? An evaluation of 3 types of memory. Sleep 2006;29:533–44.
20. Twigg GL, Papaioannou I, Jackson M, et al. Obstructive sleep apnea syndrome is associated with deficits in verbal but not visual memory. Am J Respir Crit Care Med 2010;182:98–103.
21. Beebe D, Groesz L, Wells C, et al. The neuropsychological effects of obstructive sleep apnea: a meta-analysis of norm-referenced and case-controlled data. Sleep 2003;26:298–307.

22. Wallace A, Bucks RS. Memory and obstructive sleep apnea: a meta-analysis. Sleep 2013;36(2):203–20.

23. Hoth KF, Zimmerman ME, Meschede KA, et al. Obstructive sleep apnea: impact of hypoxemia on memory. Sleep Breath 2013;17(2):811–7.

24. Kim LJ, Martinez D, Fiori CZ, et al. Hypomyelination, memory impairment, and blood-brain barrier permeability in a model of sleep apnea. Brain Res 2015;1597:28–36.

25. O'Toole M, editor. Miller-Keane encyclopedia and dictionary of medicine, nursing, and allied health. 7th edition. Camden (United Kingdom): Saunders; 2003.

26. Rouleau I, Decary A, Chicoine AJ, et al. Procedural skill learning in obstructive sleep apnea syndrome. Sleep 2002;25:401–11.

27. Aloia MS, Arnedt JT, Davis JD, et al. Neuropsychological sequelae of obstructive sleep apnea-hypopnea syndrome: a critical review. J Int Neuropsychol Soc 2004;10(5):772–85.

28. Bucks RS, Olaithe M, Eastwood P. Neurocognitive function in obstructive sleep apnoea: a meta-review. Respirology 2013;18(1):61–70.

29. Landry S, Anderson C, Andrewartha P, et al. The impact of obstructive sleep apnea on motor skill acquisition and consolidation. J Clin Sleep Med 2014;10(5):491–6.

30. Djonlagic I, Saboisky J, Carusona A, et al. Increased sleep fragmentation leads to impaired off-line consolidation of motor memories in humans. PLoS One 2012;7(3):e34106.

31. Goldstein AN, Walker MP. The role of sleep in emotional brain function. Annu Rev Clin Psychol 2014;10:679–708.

32. Beebe DW, Gozal D. Obstructive sleep apnea and the prefrontal cortex: towards a comprehensive model linking nocturnal upper airway obstruction to daytime cognitive and behavioral deficits. J Sleep Res 2002;11:1–6.

33. Lee SA, Paek JH, Han SH. REM-related sleep-disordered breathing is associated with depressive symptoms in men but not in women. Sleep Breath 2016;20:995–1002.

34. BaHammam AS, Kendzerska T, Gupta R, et al. Comorbid depression in obstructive sleep apnea: an under-recognized association. Sleep Breath 2016;20(2):447–56.

35. Garbarino S, Bardwell WA, Guglielmi O, et al. Association of anxiety and depression in obstructive sleep apnea patients: a systematic review and meta-analysis. Behav Sleep Med 2018;1–23. [Epub ahead of print].

36. Acker J, Richter K, Piehl A, et al. Obstructive sleep apnea (OSA) and clinical depression-prevalence in a sleep center. Sleep Breath 2017;21(2):311–8.

37. Lee SA, Yoon H, Kim HW. Is severe obstructive sleep apnea associated with less depressive symptoms? J Psychosom Res 2019;122:6–12.

38. Rosenzweig I, Weaver TE, Morrell MJ. Obstructive sleep apnea and the central nervous system: neural adaptive processes, cognition and performance. In: Kryger MH, Roth T, editors. Principles and practice of sleep medicine. 6th edition. Philadelphia: Elsevier; 2017. p. 1154–66.e3. Chp 117.

39. Borges JG, Ginani GE, Hachul H, et al. Executive functioning in obstructive sleep apnea syndrome patients without comorbidities: focus on the fractionation of executive functions. J Clin Exp Neuropsychol 2013;35(10):1094–107.

40. Olaithe M, Bucks RS. Executive dysfunction in OSA before and after treatment: a meta-analysis. Sleep 2013;36:1297–305.

41. Idiaquez J, Santos I, Santin J, et al. Neurobehavioral and autonomic alterations in adults with obstructive sleep apnea. Sleep Med 2014;15(11):1319–23.

42. Werli KS, Otuyama LJ, Bertolucci PH, et al. Neurocognitive function in patients with residual excessive sleepiness from obstructive sleep apnea: a prospective controlled study. Sleep Med 2016;26:6–11.

43. Yilmaz Z, Voyvoda N, Inan E, et al. Factors affecting executive functions in obstructive sleep apnea syndrome and volumetric changes in the prefrontal cortex. Springerplus 2016;5(1):1934.

44. Weichard AJ, Walter LM, Hollis SL, et al. Association between slow-wave activity, cognition and behavior in children with sleep-disordered breathing. Sleep Med 2016;25:49–55.

45. Christiansz JA, Lappin CR, Weichard AJ, et al. Slow wave activity and executive dysfunction in children with sleep disordered breathing. Sleep Breath 2018;22(2):517–25.

46. Cohen P, Alexander S, Smith T, et al. Effects of hypoxia and normocarbia on cerebral blood flow and metabolism in conscious man. J Appl Physiol 1967;23:183–9.

47. Findley LJ, Barth JT, Powers DC, et al. Cognitive impairment in patients with obstructive sleep apnea and associated hypoxemia. Chest 1986;90:686–90.

48. Blackwell T, Yaffe K, Laffan A, et al. Associations between sleep-disordered breathing, nocturnal hypoxemia, and subsequent cognitive decline in older community-dwelling men: the Osteoporotic Fractures in Men Sleep Study. J Am Geriatr Soc 2015;63(3):453–61.

49. Lim DC, Pack AI. Obstructive sleep apnea and cognitive impairment. Sleep Med Rev 2014;18(1):35–48.

50. Ward CP, McCoy JG, McKenna JT, et al. Spatial learning and memory deficits following exposure to 24 h of sleep fragmentation or intermittent hypoxia

in a rat model of obstructive sleep apnea. Brain Res 2009;1294:128–37.

51. Pilcher JJ, Huffcutt AI. Effects of sleep deprivation on performance: a meta-analysis. Sleep 1996; 19(4):318–26.

52. Lim J, Dinges DF. A meta-analysis of the impact of short-term sleep deprivation on cognitive variables. Psychol Bull 2010;136(3):375–89.

53. Kung SC, Shen YC, Chang ET, et al. Hypercapnia impaired cognitive and memory functions in obese patients with obstructive sleep apnoea. Sci Rep 2018;8(1):17551.

54. Tomfohr LM, Edwards KM, Dimsdale JE. In obstructive sleep apnea associated with cortisol levels? A systemic review of the research evidence. Sleep Med Rev 2012;16(3):243–9.

55. Kritikou I, Basta M, Vgontzas AN, et al. Sleep apnea and the hypothalamic-pituitary-adrenal axis in men and women: effects of continuous positive airway pressure. Eur Respir J 2016;47(2):531–40.

56. Edwards KM, Kamart R, Tomfohr LM, et al. Obstructive sleep apnea and neurocognitive performance: the role of cortisol. Sleep Med 2014;15(1):27–32.

57. Kushida CA, Nichols DA, Holmes TH, et al. Effects of continuous positive airway pressure on neurocognitive function in obstructive sleep apnea patients: the apnea positive pressure long-term efficacy study (APPLES). Sleep 2012;35(12):1593–602.

58. Antic NA, Catcheside P, Buchan C, et al. The effect of CPAP in normalizing daytime sleepiness, quality of life, and neurocognitive function in patients with moderate to severe OSA. Sleep 2011;34(1):111–9.

59. Richards KC, Gooneratne N, Dicicco B, et al. CPAP adherence may slow 1-year cognitive decline in older adults with mild cognitive impairment and apnea. J Am Geriatr Soc 2019;67(3):558–64.

60. Gupta A, Tripathi A, Sharma P. The long-term effects of mandibular advancement splint on cardiovascular fitness and psychomotor performance in patients with mild to moderate obstructive sleep apnea: a prospective study. Sleep Breath 2017;21:781–9.

61. Yu Y, Chen YX, Liu L, et al. Neuropsychological functioning after adenotonsillectomy in children with obstructive sleep apnea: a meta-analysis. J Huazhong Univ Sci Technolog Med Sci 2017; 37(3):453–61.

62. Woodson BT, Strohl KP, Soose RJ, et al. Upper airway stimulation for obstructive sleep apnea: 5-year outcomes. Otolaryngol Head Neck Surg 2018; 159(1):194–202.

Posttraumatic Stress Disorder, Traumatic Brain Injury, Sleep, and Performance in Military Personnel

Brian A. Moore, PhD[a,b],*, Matthew S. Brock, MD[c], Allison Brager, PhD[d], Jacob Collen, MD[e], Matthew LoPresti, PhD[f], Vincent Mysliwiec, MD[a]

KEYWORDS

- Posttraumatic stress disorder (PTSD) • Traumatic brain injury (TBI) • Sleep disorders • Performance
- Military personnel • Veterans

KEY POINTS

- Unequivocally posttraumatic stress disorder, traumatic brain injury, and disturbed sleep negatively impact the performance of military personnel; however, the magnitude of the associated performance degradation is not fully known.
- For military leaders it is paramount to address sleep disturbances because many are amenable to therapy and improvement of sleep is critical in maintaining performance.
- The inciting trauma, temporal proximity to the trauma, and comorbid disorders impact the performance in patients with posttraumatic stress disorder.
- Performance decrements associated with traumatic brain injury are typically commensurate with the severity of the injury.
- Because posttraumatic stress disorder, traumatic brain injury, and sleep disturbances are frequently comorbid, studies must evaluate the presence or absence of these disorders to determine how each disorder individually and in combination affects performance.

INTRODUCTION

Long-accepted research has shown that no act of will or ethical passion, no degree of training will preserve the ability to discriminate friend from foe, armed enemy from noncombatant, or a militarily useful target from a distraction after 96 hours of sleep deprivation.[1]

Although the need for sleep as self-care is recognized by the military, it remains at the extremes of sleep loss, as this quote highlights, whereby military leaders acknowledge performance impairments. In fact, obtaining fewer than

Disclaimer: The opinions and assertions in this article are those of the authors and do not represent those of the Department of the Air Force, Department of the Army, Department of Defense, or the U.S. Government.
[a] The University of Texas Health Science Center at San Antonio, 7550 IH 10 West, Suite 1300, San Antonio, TX 78229, USA; [b] The University of Texas at San Antonio, One UTSA Circle, San Antonio, TX 78229, USA; [c] Department of Sleep Medicine, Wilford Hall Ambulatory Surgical Center, 1100 Wilford Hall Loop Building 4554, JBSA-Lackland AFB, San Antonio, TX 78236, USA; [d] Human Performance Operations and Education Recruiting Outreach Company, United States Army Recruiting Command, Fort Knox, KY, 40121, USA; [e] Uniformed Services University of the Health Sciences, 4301 Jones Bridge Road, Bethesda, MD 20814, USA; [f] US Army Medical Research Directorate-West, Walter Reed Army Institute of Research, 9933 W. Johnson St., Joint Base Lewis-McChord, WA 98433, USA
* Corresponding author. The University of Texas at San Antonio, One UTSA Circle, San Antonio, TX 78229.
E-mail address: Mooreb6@uthscsa.edu

Sleep Med Clin 15 (2020) 87–100
https://doi.org/10.1016/j.jsmc.2019.11.004

6 hours of sleep on a regular nightly basis can negatively impact performance.[2] There is growing body of literature indicating that posttraumatic stress disorder (PTSD) and traumatic brain injury (TBI), both of which are relatively common in the active military population, can similarly impact performance. In this article, we review the literature regarding these disorders and the performance of military personnel. The concept of performance is primarily cognitive in nature, but also includes social and physical domains. Whereas the performance of military duties is impaired when these disorders are present, we describe that there is a current lack of understanding of the magnitude of the associated performance decrements. This gap is present because most performance assessments, especially in the setting of PTSD and TBI, are standardized neuropsychological tests, as opposed to the actual performance of military duties or skill relevant tasks.

POSTTRAUMATIC STRESS DISORDER

The roots of pathologic stress response syndromes can be readily identified in writings dating back thousands of years. The Assyrians, Romans, and Greeks all wrote of a disorder with no corporeal cause that would afflict their most stalwart warriors, causing them to break down into hysteria and lose their sight and the ability to speak.[3] These early descriptions provide insight into the acute complete incapacitation of a traumatized individual, whereby they had severe decrements, if not the total inability to perform their duties. In the last century, a disorder like that described in ancient cultures has been called by many names (eg, shell shock, gross stress reaction, battle stress, combat fatigue, and traumatic war neuroses). Most recently, the term posttraumatic stress disorder, or more commonly PTSD, has been used to encompass this constellation of symptoms.[4]

Although combat-related trauma and its effects on individuals have been written about for millennia, it was not until World War I that the effects of trauma exposure (psychological and physical) were systematically characterized. During the Great War, large numbers of soldiers who could no longer perform their military duties presented with symptoms of amnesia, poor concentration, headache, tinnitus, dizziness, and difficulty sleeping. Physicians noted that the symptoms manifested in a similar manner to soldiers presenting with cerebral injury and dubbed this "shell shock."[5] This disorder was poorly understood because exposure to traumatic events, lack of sleep, and physical injury were all potential reasons for a soldier's incapacitation. Shell shock was a contentious diagnosis,

especially in the absence of physical injury, and eventually became stigmatized.[6,7] Currently, it is recognized that mental disorders, to include PTSD, "are usually associated with significant distress or disability in social, occupational, or other important activities."[4] Thus, the stigma associated with what is now known as PTSD may have developed in part because afflicted soldiers were viewed as incapable of performing their duties.[8] Although our current understanding of disorders akin to shell shock (eg, PTSD and/or TBI) has substantially advanced since the initial characterizations, there is a limited understanding of the acute and chronic effects of PTSD and TBI on a soldier's ability to perform their military duties.

MILITARY TRAINING, STRESS, AND PERFORMANCE

Combat operations expose military personnel to many stressors that result in combat stress. Some military personnel respond to combat stress with an unprecedented ability for heroism and duty performance[9]; conversely, others become incapacitated and unfit for combat.[10] Although combat stress is not a diagnosis of PTSD, it is for many the precursor to this disorder with 10% to 20% of soldiers developing PTSD.[11,12] Although objective assessments of performance in actual combat operations are not available, there are studies that evaluated active duty military personnel in a number of stressful situations, including simulated prisoner of war camps,[13] survival school,[14] combat diving school, Army Rangers, and Navy Seals.[15] The findings of these studies reported that the stressful training environment, as well as symptoms of dissociation, were negatively associated with the performance of military relevant skills. The authors reported that military personnel received "little sleep,"[13] and in 1 study that the Rangers obtained 3 hours of sleep in 72 hours and 1 hour of sleep in 73 hours for the Navy Seals.[15] Near-complete lack of sleep is frequently present in combat operations. How this major factor, sleep deprivation before military or combat operations, degrades performance and/or contributes in and of itself to combat stress and increased risk of accidents and PTSD/TBI, is truly unknown but of primary importance, specifically because obtaining sleep is a defined target that can be obtained as opposed to avoiding trauma or casualties.

POSTTRAUMATIC STRESS DISORDER AND PERFORMANCE

In general, patients with PTSD report cognitive difficulties, especially attending to and recalling information.[16,17] Some memory impairments are postulated to be PTSD specific,[18] with 36% of patients with PTSD reporting some level of impaired explicit recall.[17] Conversely, these same patients often report vivid recall of prior traumatic experiences as well as trauma-related nightmares.[19] In assessing the literature regarding PTSD and performance, which includes civilian as well as veteran populations, there are variations in terms of the timing of the assessments, which has ranged from a real-time performance assessments after a stressful training exercise to formal neuropsychological testing conducted days to decades after the inciting traumatic experience; the specific tests used to evaluate performance[20,21]; and the diagnostic criteria for PTSD, which has changed since its initial presentation in the third edition of the *Diagnostic and Statistical Manual of Mental Disorders*,[22] to the current criteria in the fifth edition of the *Diagnostic and Statistical Manual of Mental Disorders*.[4] Despite the noted variances, the evidence supports that individuals with PTSD have neurocognitive deficits in overall executive functioning and verbal memory,[23] although the deficits may be subtle and vary among the population studied.[24]

In an early study assessing the cognitive performance of Vietnam Veterans with chronic PTSD, compared with those with anxiety alone and a control group with no underlying behavioral health disorder, comprehensive neuropsychological testing including the Wechsler Adult Intelligence Scale-Revised Block Design subtest, the California Verbal Learning Test, the Rey-Osterrieth Complex Figure Drawing Test, and the Paced Auditory Serial Addition Test found no significant differences in performance.[21] Similarly, LeBlanc and colleagues[25] examined the impact(s) of prior traumatic experiences and ongoing stress-related symptoms on performance in an adaptive simulated stressful training exercise in a cohort of police recruits. They found police recruits with high levels of trauma symptoms did not exhibit impairments in judgment, communication, or situational control compared with those with little to no trauma symptoms.[25]

Conversely, Esterman and colleagues[26] examined 123 veterans and found those with PTSD (most of whom had comorbid sleep disturbances) demonstrated reductions in sustained attention. Similarly, Brandes and colleagues[20] evaluated the acute effects on performance in trauma survivors (*n* = 48) and found that relative to patients with low levels of PTSD symptoms, those with higher levels had impaired attention and immediate recall for figural information as well as lower IQ scores. When the high PTSD symptom group

was compared with the low PTSD symptom group, controlling for depressive symptoms, no significant differences were present. The authors of this study concluded that a lower IQ and impaired attention were associated with both PTSD and depressive symptoms.[20] This assertion is not unique; other investigators have reported PTSD to be correlated with lower intelligence and neuroanatomic changes to include most notably smaller hippocampal volume.[27] Interestingly, in a study that evaluated women who suffered abuse as children, there were no differences in hippocampal volume or memory.[28] These contrasting findings in terms of both neuroanatomic changes and cognitive performance may emanate from the timing of the trauma to the subsequent assessment and/or to the nature of the trauma itself (ie, combat, motor vehicle accident, sexual assault) as well as if there were other factors such as sleep deprivation present preceding the traumatic event that precipitated an individual's PTSD. Another potential reason for decreased cognitive performance in PTSD is locus coeruleus dysfunction.[29] The locus coeruleus is important in maintaining focus and dysregulation of the locus coeruleus could explain some of the cognitive deficits in PTSD.[30]

A meta-analysis evaluated 60 studies that assessed neurocognitive function in PTSD and included 1779 individuals with PTSD, 1446 trauma-exposed controls, and 895 true controls.[23] The findings of this study supported significant neurocognitive deficits in PTSD with the most pronounced in verbal learning, speed of information processing, attention/working memory, and verbal memory.[23] In this article, individuals with PTSD who were treatment seeking had more pronounced deficits. More recently, a rigorous study that controlled for comorbid TBI, depression, and substance abuse evaluated neuropsychological function in veterans with PTSD compared with individuals with combat exposure without PTSD.[31] This study found that veterans with PTSD had significantly worse speed of information processing and executive functioning; however, they had no decrements in attention or working memory, verbal/language functioning, visuoconstruction, or episodic memory. Notably, the decrease in executive functioning in this study correlated with self-reported decreased occupational performance.

Other factors that may contribute to decreased performance is that military personnel and veterans with PTSD are typically male, have had combat-related trauma, and higher levels of comorbid behavioral health issues such as depression.[32] In a relatively large study of 5353 Korean War Veterans, the comorbidity of PTSD and depression was the most frequent diagnosis, followed by PTSD, and then depression alone.[33] Although this study did not directly evaluate performance, veterans with PTSD and depression had the lowest self-reported quality of life and life satisfaction. Additionally, patients with PTSD are at greater risk for maladaptive social functioning.[34] Maladaptive behaviors include an increased risk of substance abuse, suicide attempts, domestic violence, divorce, and homelessness.[35] These symptoms may in part emanate from the symptoms of PTSD as well as the fact that individuals with PTSD tend to have less social support and decreased family cohesion and life satisfaction.[36] Although the maladaptive behaviors, especially substance abuse, can negatively impact performance, our understanding of the impact of these behaviors on performance in PTSD is limited by a lack of standardized assessments used to assess social functioning and the subsequent impact on an individual's performance.[34]

Regarding work performance, there are some studies that have reported that individuals who suffer from PTSD are less productive, work fewer hours, and use more sick days compared with individuals without PTSD. One study assessed 325 Vietnam Veterans who received treatment for PTSD; in this study, individuals with more severe PTSD symptoms were more likely to work part time or not at all.[37,38] Thus, it would be reasonable to equate this decreased ability to work full time associated with PTSD and PTSD symptoms as a decrease in the overall performance of an individual. To date, the quantifiable impacts of PTSD (eg, cognitive, physical, socioeconomic, or task specific) on an individual's actual duty performance are insufficiently evaluated. The decrement in performance seems to vary in the acute versus chronic state of PTSD. Further, the actual performance impairment is further complicated by the frequent presence of comorbid disorders, which can further negatively impact performance.

TRAUMATIC BRAIN INJURY AND PERFORMANCE

TBIs occur after trauma that induces structural injury or physiologic disruption to normal brain functioning.[39] The standard practice and diagnostic guidelines for the management of TBI classify each by severity, namely, as mild, moderate, or severe.[40] It is worth clarifying that mild TBI, concussion, mild head trauma, and mild head injury are frequently used interchangeably.[41] For this article, we use mild TBI to address these differences in terminology. The most frequently diagnosed severity of TBI is mild TBI, followed by

moderate and severe TBIs (82.3%, 9.7%, and 1%, respectively).[42] Individuals who experience a mild TBI frequently report acute symptoms such as dizziness, nausea, difficulties sleeping, reduced attention, amnesia, or headache,[42,43] as well as other cognitive deficits such as memory acquisition, slowed processing speed, issues multitasking, losing train of one's thoughts, and global cognitive functioning.[41] In mild TBI, symptoms typically manifest within 24 hours after the injury[41] and resolve without medical attention in approximately 7 days.[44–51]

Recent studies report TBI to be a persistent concern for active duty military personnel.[42,52,53] This is largely due to the nature of the contemporary operating environment. Specifically, military personnel are at increased risk of exposure to a number of circumstances that may be related to TBI ,including rocket-propelled grenades, artillery, and blast exposure from improvised explosive devices. A RAND survey completed in 2008 reported data from initial waves of military personnel involved in the troop surge to Iraq in 2006 and found that nearly 20% experienced a mild TBI during deployment.[35] A separate study by Swanson and colleagues[39] reported similar rates nearly 10 years later. A more recent report by the Defense and Veterans Brain Injury Center identified 383,947 cases of TBI diagnosed in the Department of Defense since 2000.[42] Although TBI is prevalent among military personnel, approximately 10 million cases are recorded annually among the global populace, primarily owing to car accidents or sporting events.[54] As such, a large portion of the extant literature on TBI and performance is derived from sports medicine[43] with civilian patients. For this reason, the present section addresses the acute and long-term performance decrements in both civilians and military personnel.

TRAUMATIC BRAIN INJURY IMPACTS ON PERFORMANCE IN ATHLETES AND OTHER CIVILIANS

A seminal study of athletes with a history of TBI followed 79 college football players over the course of 90 days.[48] This study found that, relative to non-TBI controls, those with a mild TBI displayed higher levels of cognitive impairment and balance problems immediately after experiencing the mild TBI, but most symptoms resolved within 7 days. Specifically, mild cognitive impairments improved to baseline levels within 5 to 7 days and balance impairments resolved within 3 to 5 days.[48] In their sample, McCrea and colleagues[48] found no significant differences in functional impairments between the controls and participants with a mild

TBI at 90 days. Other studies that assessed concussed athletes at 1, 3, and 5 days after injury have shown similar findings with mild deficits in balance, concentration, working memory, immediate memory recall, and rapid visual processing after injury.[55] A meta-analysis of 21 studies evaluated the neuropsychological impact of sports-related mild TBI on athletes and found within the first 24 hours to 7 days after injury, there were decrements in delayed memory, memory acquisition, and global cognitive functioning.[45] When considering the results of 21 studies, however, Belanger and Vanderploeg[45] determined that within 7 to 10 days after the injury the overall cognitive performance of participants with a TBI did not differ from noninjured control subjects. It is important to note there is no established acute period of symptoms related to a TBI; the literature broadly discusses acute impacts of TBI as occurring within 7 days after the injury.

Chronic cognitive deficits associated with TBI are known to interfere in nearly every aspect of daily living, including work, relationships, and leisure activities.[56] These cognitive deficits contribute to impaired performance, primarily in areas such as disorganized memory encoding[57,58] and deficits in executive functioning,[57] attentional focus,[59,60] planning, and decision making.[61,62] Numerous studies have reported when post-TBI symptoms persist beyond 3 to 6 months, individuals are also more likely to develop vocational disabilities. For instance, Sinopoli and colleagues[63] recently examined a cohort of 13 individuals with a history of mild TBI at 3 and 6 months after injury. Compared with a noninjured control group, the participants with a history of mild TBI performed slower on tasks that required working memory and dual tasking. In line with this, a sample of 111 individuals with TBI showed significant deficits 1-year after injury related to executive functioning, rather than speed of processing or memory.[64] Recently, Nelson and colleagues[65] examined 1154 individuals who sustained a mild TBI and were treated at 11 separate US level I trauma centers. In all, they found that functional impairments were most severe at 2 weeks after injury, but that 53% of the study participants reported persistent functional impairments at 12 months after injury with 17% reporting work-related and social functioning difficulties.

In regard to the dynamic relationship between TBI and performance, specific considerations must be given to the severity and manifest symptoms, the environment,[66] or mode[67] by which a TBI is sustained (eg, blast related vs blunt force), and the effected neuroanatomic regions. The exact physiologic mechanisms by which TBI

impacts performance are not fully elucidated; yet, it is known that TBIs frequently impact the frontal lobes and circuitry[68] and a major factor influencing the impact of TBI on performance is the severity of the injury. Moderate and severe TBIs frequently result in more severe and chronic cognitive deficits (eg, decrements in awareness, reasoning, language, visuospatial processing, and general intelligence) than mild TBI.[45]

There are a number of factors related to a mild TBI that can determine if an individual develops long-term performance decrements to include single versus multiple mild TBI, age, and acute symptomatology. In the majority of individuals, an isolated mild TBI is unlikely to cause persistent cognitive deficits.[69,70] Repeated injuries, however, pose an increased risk of long-term cognitive deficits.[71–73] In some of these studies, repeated injuries were found to have a dose–response relationship whereby more injuries resulted in greater cognitive performance deficits. Further supporting the long-term consequences of multiple mild TBIs is a meta-analysis of 21 studies that found athletes with multiple mild TBIs were nearly 8 times more likely to exhibit decreased performance in memory tasks relative to athletes who had never sustained a mild TBI.[45]

Age at time of injury has also been shown to influence the chronicity of TBI symptoms, whereby younger individuals seem to be more susceptible to long-term cognitive deficits. Lah and colleagues[74] examined 14 children who had sustained a severe TBI during childhood and found that severe TBI impacts both explicit and implicit memory, specifically in children who sustained a TBI early in life (<6 years of age). A meta-analysis of 6 studies examining time to recovery between high school and collegiate athletes with mild TBI found recovery times for cognitive impairments were roughly equal between the 2 groups (7 days vs 5 days, respectively), but that high school athletes took 2.5 times longer (15 days vs 6 days) to report feeling asymptomatic.[75] Numerous other studies have examined the impacts of mild TBI symptoms on recovery. One study of 107 high school football players with a history of mild TBI found that individuals who reported immediate feelings of dizziness were 6.3 times more likely to have a prolonged period of recovery (eg, ≥3 weeks).[76] In another study, McCrea and colleagues[47] examined 570 athletes with mild TBI, reporting that acute onset symptoms to include loss of consciousness and amnesia were related to a prolonged mild TBI symptomatology. Similarly, a study of 139 prisoners with a history of TBI found the severity of a sustained TBI negatively correlated with intellectual performance such that intellectual functioning was poorer among the sample with a TBI and observed performance was commensurate with the severity of the injury.[77] In all, the preponderance of evidence in athletes and civilians shows mild TBI results in acute impaired cognitive performance[45] as well as neurologic symptoms, which could impair performance in the majority of individuals.

TRAUMATIC BRAIN INJURY IMPACTS ON PERFORMANCE IN THE MILITARY

The impact of TBI on the performance of military duties is not as well understood as the acute neurocognitive deficits in civilians. A recently completed systematic review of 31 military-related TBI studies reported inconsistent findings surrounding long-term impacts of TBI, frequent methodologic shortcomings, and substantial variation in measurement approaches among the reviewed studies.[78] Numerous studies have indicated a key limitation to interpreting the impacts of TBI in military personnel is the confounding factor of behavioral health concerns.[78–83] For instance, between 33% and 65% of veterans with TBI also report PTSD symptoms.[84–87] A separate systematic review of 13 articles identified only 3 that were deemed to be at low risk of bias[88] and acceptable for analysis. This study found that military personnel with mild TBI frequently have PTSD symptoms. It also concluded that although there was a slight decrease in neurocognitive performance in patients with mild TBI, it was within the realm of normal cognition. Conversely, Boyle and colleagues[88] identified only limited evidence supporting the supposition that behavioral health issues impact recovery and prognosis after mild TBI.

A seminal study conducted by Luethcke and colleagues[89] examined 82 forward-deployed military personnel who met criteria for a mild TBI (n = 42 non–blast-related injury and n = 40 blast-related injury) within 72 hours. Using computerized neurocognitive testing, clinical interviews, and a battery of subjective measures, they found the groups did not significantly differ in terms of alterations in consciousness, somatic symptoms, concentration impairment, or sleep disturbances.[89] However, immediately after the injury, postural stability was impacted more in the nonblast cohort, whereas hearing deficiencies were more frequent in the blast group.[89] Although they did not find significant differences between the groups in cognitive performance on the Automated Neuropsychological Assessment Metrics subtests, test performance inversely correlated with duration of loss of consciousness.

Interestingly, Luethcke and colleagues[89] also did not note any differences in PTSD or insomnia symptoms, or psychological symptoms between the 2 groups. This finding may have been related to the temporal proximity of the comprehensive evaluation as opposed to nearly all other studies, which performed the evaluation months to years after the initial injury.

The literature has shown that, regardless of etiology, acute symptoms of psychological distress related to combat may cause higher rates of perceived cognitive dysfunction than is solely due to a mild TBI.[78,90] Specifically, Brickell and colleagues[90] examined 101 military personnel with a history of TBI and found long-term neurocognitive performance to be unrelated to postinjury levels of executive function. Rather, they asserted that subjective symptoms of executive dysfunction were more strongly related to psychological distress than objective observations.[90] A larger study by Mortera and colleagues[91] found 236 veterans with a history of TBI had high pain levels, irritability, sleep disturbances, forgetfulness, and headaches. Additionally, nearly 40% of this sample reported poor performance in the domain of productivity. The authors attributed this finding to high rates of comorbid depression.[91] Another study compared groups of military personnel who were within 6 months of having a TBI (mild TBI, n = 41; moderate TBI, n = 42) and found no significant differences between groups on measures of neurocognitive functioning.[92] Lange and colleagues[92] reported that military personnel with an uncomplicated mild TBI had significantly higher levels of anxiety and aggression than military personnel who experienced a complicated mild TBI. Similarly, a series of studies examined 249 veterans with a history of TBI. In this study the veterans who rated their TBI sequelae as very severe were more likely to put forth suboptimal efforts on objective testing.[93] In total, these findings further substantiate the impact of both diagnosed and undiagnosed behavioral health disorders on the combined performance decrements in military personnel and veterans.

Studies of military personnel have also reported findings similar to those found in the civilian literature. For instance, numerous cases of military personnel with repeated head injuries have shown advanced instances of chronic traumatic encephalopathy.[94–96] Clinically, chronic traumatic encephalopathy is recognized as a progressive neurodegenerative disease[97] that presents with behavioral changes, executive dysfunction, memory loss, and cognitive impairments.[98] There is a series of case studies involving 5 military personnel who experienced multiple concussions.

This study found evidence of early-onset chronic traumatic encephalopathy as well as PTSD in the service members.[98] Because some TBIs can result in long-term neurologic concerns, it is unsurprising that the systematic review by O'Neil and colleagues[78] found approximately 20% of veterans with a history of TBI reported issues integrating into the civilian workforce. Other studies have reported long-term impairments in the social domain to include developing friendships as well as decreased satisfaction with and quality of life.[99,100] However, not all research supports long-term sequelae related to TBI. A study of 907 soldiers with a TBI by Terrio and colleagues[101] found that symptoms related to TBI, primarily headaches and dizziness, subsided over time with no long-term decrements in performance.

One of the challenges in assessing the impact of TBI on performance is a lack of validity in standardized approaches[102] or consensus on how the assessment of TBI should be performed. A common method is focusing on symptom-based outcomes such as the resolution of postconcussion syndrome.[103] This approach is limited because TBI symptoms are primarily subjective and many are nonspecific and can occur with medical and behavioral medicine disorders.[104] Other TBI research has looked at the structural impact of acute and chronic TBI using sophisticated neuroimaging techniques.[105] Although useful, functional neuroimaging gives little information about performance, remains largely exploratory, and therefore is not practical for all patients with TBI. Questionnaires and neuropsychological testing are commonly used to assess individuals after TBI, but even these do not necessarily translate into a performance assessment that can determine the patient's ability to perform at work, on the field, or on the battlefield. A standardized assessment of performance after injury at set time points is needed to aid in prognostication after TBI as well as the development of outcomes-based prevention and treatment strategies.

SLEEP AND PERFORMANCE

It is widely accepted that initial military training, even at elite military academies,[106,107] is characterized by highly demanding physical and academic training loads in the setting of insufficient sleep. Beyond initial entry training, 2 large-scale studies found that 72% and 69% of military personnel report sleeping fewer than 6 hours per night,[108,109] with the number of combat exposures and combat-related injuries being strong predictors of even shorter sleep duration, that is, less than 5 hours per night. In the most recent population-based survey of sleep collected during Operation Enduring Freedom, 57% of 6118 military personnel reported highly disrupted sleep with the severity dependent on mission type (eg, day vs night operations) and number of deployments.[110] Thus, insufficient and disrupted sleep is normative and pervasive across a service member's career.

Military personnel have nonstandard shift work schedules, routinely participate in sustained operations that are more than 24 hours in duration, distributed operations greater than 12 hours in duration across several days or weeks, and work in austere environments. These occupational requirements manifest in total sleep deprivation (TSD), chronic sleep restriction (CSR), misaligned internal sleep/wake rhythms with environmental rhythms (ie, circadian misalignment), and sleep fragmentation.[111] Further, the consolidated and restorative sleep that is required to perform optimally in physically and mentally demanding military operations is rarely achieved. Thus, despite austere environmental conditions and suboptimal sleeping conditions, the high physiologic drive to sleep owing to acute and chronic insufficient sleep is one of many reasons military personnel are stereotyped for being able to sleep at any given opportunity.

There is a rich body of evidence showing direct change, largely decline, in psychophysiologic performance with sleep loss. The rate of decline in performance with sleep loss and return of performance to baseline levels varies with TSD (sustained operations) and CSR (distributed operations) for both simple (ie, reaction time) and complex (ie, creativity) cognitive domains.[112] For example, although tasks requiring vigilance and mathematical addition and subtraction show a dose–response curve in decline with consecutive hours of sleep lost under TSD, performance can recover to baseline levels within a single night of adequate recovery sleep.[113,114] Regarding cognitive performance under CSR, although there are dose–response deficits in performance for every night of insufficient sleep (<5 hours sleep per night), it is rare that performance recovers to baseline levels within a single night of adequate recovery sleep. In some cases, and depending on the nature of sleep loss, recovery in performance can extend for more than 7 days.[113,115] Further, recent brain imaging studies have shown via beta-amyloid deposition in the brain that neurophysiologic health minimally recovers after sleep loss, both for TSD and CSR.[116] The studies of TSD and CSR conducted in military science laboratories have additionally discovered that the rate of cognitive decline under TSD and CSR is trait dependent, with select individuals showing more stable performance (relative to baseline levels) under sleep loss (ie, termed resilient) compared with select individuals showing immediate and continual decline under sleep loss (ie, termed sensitive).[117,118]

Sleep fragmentation and subsequent sleep inertia (delayed transition from a state of sleep to high levels of alertness owing to environmental disruption) are also cause for concern for military performance. A recent study determined that higher-order performance decreases quickly and recovers slowly during episodically brief interruptions of deep (restorative) sleep, similar to episodically short total sleep durations.[119] Further, sleep inertia experienced in the middle of a nighttime sleep episode results in cognitive decline comparable to 24-hour TSD, reaching a zenith when the biological drive to sleep in the early morning hours is greatest.[120,121] Because sleep inertia is an operationally significant issue, military researchers evaluated the impact of caffeine gum to ameliorate this condition.[122] Interestingly, 100 mg of caffeine gum was found to decrease sleep inertia's effects at both 0100 and 0600 in otherwise healthy individuals.

The extrapolation of testing and evaluating psychophysiologic domains of military performance in military sciences laboratories to actual, operational performance is complex. First, psychophysiologic decline during combat operations is largely confounded by environmental stressors of heat, dehydration, and malnourishment.[123] However, not even a high-energy diet can protect against psychophysiologic decline after more than 3 days of CSR,[124] indicating that a loss of combat effectiveness is inevitable with sleep loss. In fact, 2 separate studies of combat effectiveness measured against objectively reported sleep time in a previous (Gulf War) and current (Afghanistan) military conflict found that performance degraded by 15% to 25% for every nighttime sleep duration of less than 7 hours per night. Nighttime sleep durations of less than 4 hours resulted in total combat effectiveness of 15%.[125,126] Increases in mistakes and decreased mental acuity in high-risk military environments (eg, crewmen in a nuclear reactor department) have also been reported.[127] Another important aspect of military operations is moral reasoning. In a simulated training environment where officer candidates obtained 2.5 hours of sleep per 24 hours over days, they had substantially impaired ability to conduct mature and principally oriented moral reasoning.[128] Thus, the ramifications of sleep loss on the performance of military personnel are

substantial and inversely correlated with total sleep time.

To dissect how psychophysiologic attributes at the individual level contribute to a loss of combat effectiveness at the group level under sleep loss (both TSD and CSR), most of the data, particularly for CSR studies, derive from military-relevant rather than military populations: athletes, healthcare professionals, and law enforcement. However, several parallels can be drawn from the tactical responsibilities of military personnel and sport-specific and occupational-specific schedules and psychophysiologic demands of these military-relevant populations. Each profession requires high degrees of vigilance, decision making, and emotional valence for cognitive domains and endurance, power, hand–eye coordination, and agility for physical domains. Similar to military personnel, the number of self-reported sleep complaints reaching a clinical threshold and requiring follow-up sleep consultation is indeed pervasive in collegiate athletes; reaching as high as 66% (Burke TM, Maguire K, Skeiky L, et al. Characterizing Sleep and Chronobiology in College Football Athletes. J Strength Cond Res. [Under review]).[129] Although TSD is less common for athletes, CSR in athletes is associated with more than sports-related injuries,[130] leading to reductions in cardiorespiratory capacities,[131] anaerobic power,[132] poor choice reaction time,[133] and increased confusion.[134]

There are a few studies of TSD in military populations that show the salient impact on broad domains of psychophysiologic performance. In general, the impact of TSD on the cognitive versus physical performance attributes of sustained operations, such as cardiovascular strain and tasks of divided attention, are not mutually exclusive.[135] The impact of sleep loss can be lessened to an extent through pre-exercise napping[136] of varying durations.[137] Further, the amount of cardiovascular strain during sustained endurance operations (ie, >96-hour ultra-endurance race) can modulate the degree of cognitive processing.[138] Even if cognitive performance is decreased under sleep loss, cognitive performance can still be optimized in these extreme environments by means of maintaining less than 50% maximal cardiovascular output. In a study evaluating marksmanship (a core military skill) increasing cognitive load while having restricted sleep periods further worsened performance.[139] From these studies, it is apparent that not only decreased sleep periods but also the physical and cognitive loads can synergistically decrease performance.

When delineating the impact of TSD on physical performance attributes of sustained operations, the impact is readily apparent. Studies in military personnel have reported significant declines in submaximal performance,[140] increased latency to neuromuscular fatigue, and loss of power as well as anthropometric changes with greater than 24 hours of continuous sleep loss.[141] Interestingly, the rate of decline in the speed of individual cognitive processing during sustained military operations has been reported to be more robust, showing minimal to modest declines with 36 to 72 hours of (survival) training, respectively.[142,143] However, one remarkable observation is that in both of these studies, the modest (rather than rapid decline) in cognitive processing did not return to optimal/baseline levels after military training,[142,143] pointing once again to the operational significance of adequate sleep.

SUMMARY

Sleep disturbances, PTSD, and TBI are all highly prevalent in military personnel and veterans. These conditions often overlap, are interrelated, and result in impaired performance. Insufficient sleep leads to nearly immediate and pervasive increases in physiologic and psychological stress, brain inflammation, and cortisol over-reactivity. Collectively, these physiologic and psychological states can contribute to comorbidities with PTSD and TBI owing to decreased resiliency and neuroprotection. From a performance standpoint, appropriate levels of sleep may serve to mitigate risk and maintain performance in military personnel. For years, the prevailing culture in the military favored sleep deprivation as a means of demonstrating mental and physical toughness.[107] Currently, the military is in a position to change cultural attitudes about sleep. As with their civilian counterparts, military leaders are becoming increasingly aware of the impact of sleep loss and sleep disorders on the health, safety, and performance of service members. In recent years, military branches have published doctrine on sleep and well-being, such as *The Leader's Guide to Soldier Health and Fitness* developed by the Office of the Army Surgeon General (ATP 6–22.5) that must be adopted by senior leadership while engaging in training and mission planning. Additional measures facilitating this culture shift include the development of a comprehensive, individualized sleep and alertness management system to optimize performance after sleep loss as well as the inclusion of sleep with exercise and nutrition in the US Army's Performance Triad public health campaign.[111,144]

Ensuring adequate, quality sleep in military personnel is paramount for the health and safety of service members and the success of routine and sustained operations both stateside and abroad. An understanding of how military-specific stressors contribute to the development of disturbed sleep and sleep disorders is required to develop novel individualized, effective strategies to combat poor sleep in this critical population. Further research on the relationship between disturbed sleep, PTSD, and TBI and their impact on the performance of military personnel, especially their ability to adequately perform their duties, is required.

DISCLOSURE

This research did not receive any specific grant from funding agencies in the public, commercial, or not-for-profit sectors.

REFERENCES

1. Shay J. Ethical standing for commander self-care: the need for sleep. Parameters 1998;28(2):93–105.
2. Alhola P, Polo-Kantola P. Sleep deprivation: impact on cognitive performance. Neuropsychiatr Dis Treat 2007;3(5):553–67.
3. Abdul-hamid WK, Hughes JH. Nothing new under the sun: post-traumatic stress disorders in the ancient world. Early Sci Med 2014;19(6):549–57.
4. Diagnostic and statistical manual of mental disorders: DSM-5. Arlington (VA): American Psychiatric Association; 2013.
5. Turner WA. Cases of nervous and mental shock observed in the base hospitals in France. J R Army Med Corps 1915;24:343–52.
6. Jones E, Fear NT, Wessely S. Shell shock and mild traumatic brain injury: a historical review. Am J Psychiatry 2007;164(11):1641–5.
7. Crocq MA, Crocq L. From shell shock and war neurosis to posttraumatic stress disorder: a history of psychotraumatology. Dialogues Clin Neurosci 2000;2(1):47–55.
8. Riggs DS, Mallonee S. Barriers to care for the complex presentation of Post-traumatic Stress Disorder and other post-combat psychological injuries. Handbook of Military Psychology. Springer International Publishing; 2017.
9. Bonanno GA. Loss, trauma, and human resilience: have we underestimated the human capacity to thrive after extremely aversive events? Am Psychol 2004;59(1):20–8.
10. Moore BA, Mason ST, Crow BE. Assessment and management of acute combat stress on the battlefield. In: Kennedy CH, Zillmer E, editors. Military psychology: clinical and operational applications. Guilford Press; 2012. p. 73–92.
11. Hoge CW, Riviere LA, Wilk JE, et al. The prevalence of post-traumatic stress disorder (PTSD) in US

combat soldiers: a head-to-head comparison of DSM-5 versus DSM-IV-TR symptom criteria with the PTSD checklist. Lancet Psychiatry 2014;1(4): 269–77.

12. Kok BC, Herrell RK, Thomas JL, et al. Posttraumatic stress disorder associated with combat service in Iraq or Afghanistan: reconciling prevalence differences between studies. J Nerv Ment Dis 2012;200(5):444–50.

13. Eid J, Morgan CA. Dissociation, hardiness, and performance in military cadets participating in survival training. Mil Med 2006;171(5):436–42.

14. Morgan CA, Doran A, Steffian G, et al. Stress-induced deficits in working memory and visuoconstructive abilities in Special Operations soldiers. Biol Psychiatry 2006;60(7):722–9.

15. Lieberman HR, Bathalon GP, Falco CM, et al. The fog of war: decrements in cognitive performance and mood associated with combat-like stress. Aviat Space Environ Med 2005;76(7 Suppl):C7–14.

16. McNally RJ, Frueh BC. Why are Iraq and Afghanistan War Veterans seeking PTSD disability compensation at unprecedented rates? J Anxiety Disord 2013;27(5):520–6.

17. Hart J, Kimbrell T, Fauver P, et al. Cognitive dysfunctions associated with PTSD: evidence from World War II prisoners of war. J Neuropsychiatry Clin Neurosci 2008;20(3):309–16.

18. Danckwerts A, Leathem J. Questioning the link between PTSD and cognitive dysfunction. Neuropsychol Rev 2003;13(4):221–35.

19. Wolfe J, Schlesinger LK. Performance of PTSD patients on standard tests of memory. Implications for trauma. Ann N Y Acad Sci 1997;821:208–18.

20. Brandes D, Ben-schachar G, Gilboa A, et al. PTSD symptoms and cognitive performance in recent trauma survivors. Psychiatry Res 2002;110(3): 231–8.

21. Zalewski C, Thompson W, Gottesman I. Comparison of neuropsychological test performance in PTSD, generalized anxiety disorder, and control Vietnam veterans. Assessment 1994;1(2): 133–42.

22. The diagnostic and statistical manual of mental disorders. 3rd edition. Washington, DC: American Psychiatric Association; 1980.

23. Scott JC, Matt GE, Wrocklage KM, et al. A quantitative meta-analysis of neurocognitive functioning in posttraumatic stress disorder. Psychol Bull 2015;141(1):105–40.

24. Newman J, Marmar C. Executive function in posttraumatic stress disorder. In: Executive functions in health and disease, 20. Academic Press; 2017. p. 487–524.

25. Leblanc VR, Regehr C, Jelley RB, et al. Does posttraumatic stress disorder (PTSD) affect performance? J Nerv Ment Dis 2007;195(8):701–4.

26. Esterman M, Fortenbaugh FC, Pierce ME, et al. Trauma-related psychiatric and behavioral conditions are uniquely associated with sustained attention dysfunction. Neuropsychology 2019;33(5): 711–24.

27. O'Doherty DC, Chitty KM, Saddiqui S, et al. A systematic review and meta-analysis of magnetic resonance imaging measurement of structural volumes in posttraumatic stress disorder. Psychiatry Res 2015;232(1):1–33.

28. Pederson CL, Maurer SH, Kaminski PL, et al. Hippocampal volume and memory performance in a community-based sample of women with posttraumatic stress disorder secondary to child abuse. J Trauma Stress 2004;17(1):37–40.

29. Pietrzak RH, Gallezot JD, Ding YS, et al. Association of posttraumatic stress disorder with reduced in vivo norepinephrine transporter availability in the locus coeruleus. JAMA Psychiatry 2013; 70(11):1199–205.

30. Aston-Jones G, Rajkowski J, Cohen J. Role of locus coeruleus in attention and behavioral flexibility. Biol Psychiatry 1999;46(9):1309–20.

31. Wrocklage KM, Schweinsburg BC, Krystal JH, et al. Neuropsychological functioning in veterans with posttraumatic stress disorder: associations with performance validity, comorbidities, and functional outcomes. J Int Neuropsychol Soc 2016; 22(4):399–411.

32. Polak AR, Witteveen AB, Reitsma JB, et al. The role of executive function in posttraumatic stress disorder: a systematic review. J Affect Disord 2012; 141(1):11–21.

33. Ikin JF, Creamer MC, Sim MR, et al. Comorbidity of PTSD and depression in Korean War Veterans: prevalence, predictors, and impairment. J Affect Disord 2010;125(1–3):279–86.

34. Frueh BC, Turner SM, Beidel DC, et al. Assessment of social functioning in combat Veterans with PTSD. Aggress Violent Behav 2001;6(1):79–90.

35. Tanielian T, Jaycox LH. Invisible wounds of war psychological and cognitive injuries, their consequences, and services to assist recovery: summary. Santa Monica, (CA): RAND Corporation; 2008.

36. Tsai J, Harpaz-rotem I, Pietrzak RH, et al. The role of coping, resilience, and social support in mediating the relation between PTSD and social functioning in Veterans returning from Iraq and Afghanistan. Psychiatry 2012;75(2):135–49.

37. Smith MW, Schnurr PP, Rosenheck RA. Employment outcomes and PTSD symptom severity. Ment Health Serv Res 2005;7(2):89–101.

38. Stergiopoulos E, Cimo A, Cheng C, et al. Interventions to improve work outcomes in work-related PTSD: a systematic review. BMC Public Health 2011;11:838.

39. Swanson TM, Isaacson BM, Cyborski CM, et al. Traumatic brain injury incidence, clinical overview, and policies in the US Military Health System since 2000. Public Health Rep 2017;132(2):251–9.

40. Management of Concussion/mTBI Working Group. VA/DoD clinical practice guideline for management of concussion/mild traumatic brain injury. J Rehabil Res Dev 2009;46(6):CP1-68.

41. Prince C, Bruhns ME. Evaluation and treatment of mild traumatic brain injury: the role of neuropsychology. Brain Sci 2017;7(8).

42. Defense and Veterans Brain Injury Center (DVBIC). DoD worldwide numbers for TBI. Website. Available at: https://dvbic.dcoe.mil/system/files/tbi-numbers/worldwide-totals-2000-2018Q1-total_jun-21-2018_v1.0_2018-07-26_0.pdf. Accessed August 5, 2019.

43. Ling H, Hardy J, Zetterberg H. Neurological consequences of traumatic brain injuries in sports. Mol Cell Neurosci 2015;66(Part B):114–22.

44. Carroll LJ, Cassidy JD, Peloso PM, et al. Prognosis for mild traumatic brain injury: results of the who collaborating centre task force on mild traumatic brain injury. J Rehabil Med 2004;36(Supplement 43):84–105.

45. Belanger H, Vanderploeg R. The neuropsychological impact of sports-related concussion: a meta-analysis. J Int Neuropsychol Soc 2005;11(4):345–57.

46. Hoge CW, McGurk D, Thomas JL, et al. Mild traumatic brain injury in US soldiers returning from Iraq. N Engl J Med 2008;358(5):453–63.

47. McCrea M, Guskiewicz K, Randolph C, et al. Incidence, clinical course, and predictors of prolonged recovery time following sport-related concussion in high school and college athletes. J Int Neuropsychol Soc 2013;19(1):22–33.

48. McCrea M, Guskiewicz KM, Marshall SW, et al. Acute effects and recovery time following concussion in collegiate football players: the NCAA Concussion Study. JAMA 2003;290(19):2556–63.

49. Lee YM, Odom MJ, Zuckerman SL, et al. Does age affect symptom recovery after sports-related concussion? A study of high school and college athletes. J Neurosurg Pediatr 2013;12(6):537–44.

50. Erlanger D, Kaushik T, Cantu R, et al. Symptom-based assessment of the severity of a concussion. J Neurosurg 2003;98(3):477–84.

51. Zuckerman SL, Kuhn A, Dewan MC, et al. Structural brain injury in sports-related concussion. Neurosurg Focus 2012;33(6):E6, 1–12.

52. Institute of Medicine. Gulf war and health: volume 9: long-term effects of blast exposures. Washington, DC: The National Academies Press; 2014.

53. Okie S. Traumatic brain injury in the war zone. N Engl J Med 2005;352(20):2043–7.

54. World Health Organization. Neurological disorders: public health challenges. Geneva, Switzerland: WHO press. Available at: https://www.who.int/mental_health/neurology/neurological_disorders_report_web.pdf. Accessed July 5, 2019.

55. Guskiewicz KM, Ross SE, Marshall SW. Postural stability and neuropsychological deficits after concussion in collegiate athletes. J Athl Train 2001;36(3):263–73.

56. Rabinowitz AR, Levin HS. Cognitive sequelae of traumatic brain injury. Psychiatr Clin North Am 2014;37(1):1–11.

57. Dikmen SS, Corrigan JD, Levin HS, et al. Cognitive outcome following traumatic brain injury. J Head Trauma Rehabil 2009;24(6):430–8.

58. Levin HS, Mattis S, Ruff RM, et al. Neurobehavioral outcome following minor head injury: a three-center study. J Neurosurg 1987;66:234–43.

59. Dockree PM, Kelly SP, Roche RA, et al. Behavioural and physiological impairments of sustained attention after traumatic brain injury. Brain Res Cogn Brain Res 2004;20(3):403–14.

60. Stuss DT, Alexander MP. Executive functions and the frontal lobes: a conceptual view. Psychol Res 2000;63(3–4):289–98.

61. Malkki H. Traumatic brain injury: impaired medical decision-making capacity in TBI. Nat Rev Neurol 2016;12(10):555.

62. Sood N, Godfrey C, Anderson V, et al. Rehabilitation of executive function in pediatric traumatic brain injury (REPeaT): protocol for a randomized controlled trial for treating working memory and decision-making. BMC Pediatr 2018;18(1):362.

63. Sinopoli KJ, Chen JK, Wells G, et al. Imaging "brain strain" in youth athletes with mild traumatic brain injury during dual-task performance. J Neurotrauma 2014;31(22):1843–59.

64. Spitz G, Ponsford JL, Rudzki D, et al. Association between cognitive performance and functional outcome following traumatic brain injury: a longitudinal multilevel examination. Neuropsychology 2012;26(5):604–12.

65. Nelson LD, Temkin NR, Dikmen S, et al. Recovery after mild traumatic brain injury in patients presenting to US level I trauma centers: a transforming research and clinical knowledge in traumatic brain injury (TRACK-TBI) study. JAMA Neurol 2019;76(9):1049–59.

66. Baldassarre M, Smith B, Harp J, et al. Exploring the relationship between mild traumatic brain injury exposure and the presence and severity of postconcussive symptoms among Veterans deployed to Iraq and Afghanistan. PM R 2015;7(8):845–58.

67. Mendez MF, Owens EM, Reza-berenji G, et al. Mild traumatic brain injury from primary blast vs. blunt forces: post-concussion consequences and

functional neuroimaging. NeuroRehabilitation 2013;32(2):397–407.

68. Ponsford JL, Parcell DL, Sinclair KL, et al. Changes in sleep patterns following traumatic brain injury: a controlled study. Neurorehabil Neural Repair 2013; 27(7):613–21.

69. Savica R, Parisi JE, Wold LE, et al. High school football and risk of neurodegeneration: a community-based study. Mayo Clin Proc 2012;87: 335–40.

70. Janssen PH, Mandrekar J, Mielke MM, et al. High school football and late-life risk of neurodegenerative syndromes, 1956-1970. Mayo Clin Proc 2017; 92:66–71.

71. Guskiewicz KM, Marshall SW, Bailes J, et al. Association between recurrent concussion and late-life cognitive impairment in retired professional football players. Neurosurgery 2005;57:719–26.

72. Randolph C, Karantzoulis S, Guskiewicz K. Prevalence and characterization of mild cognitive impairment in retired national football league players. J Int Neuropsychol Soc 2013;19(8):873–80.

73. Manley G, Gardner AJ, Schneider KJ, et al. A systematic review of potential long-term effects of sport-related concussion. Br J Sports Med 2017;51(12):969–77.

74. Lah S, Epps A, Levick W, et al. Implicit and explicit memory outcome in children who have sustained severe traumatic brain injury: impact of age at injury (preliminary findings). Brain Inj 2011;25(1): 44–52.

75. Williams RM, Puetz TW, Giza CC, et al. Concussion recovery time among high school and collegiate athletes: a systematic review and meta-analysis. Sports Med 2015;45(6):893–903.

76. Lau BC, Kontos AP, Collins MW, et al. Which on-field signs/symptoms predict protracted recovery from sport-related concussion among high school football players? Am J Sports Med 2011;39(11): 2311–8.

77. Pitman I, Haddlesey C, Ramos SD, et al. The association between neuropsychological performance and self-reported traumatic brain injury in a sample of adult male prisoners in the UK. Neuropsychol Rehabil 2015;25(5):763–79.

78. O'Neil ME, Carlson K, Storzbach D, et al. Complications of mild traumatic brain injury in veterans and military personnel: a systematic review. Washington, DC: Department of Veterans Affairs (US); 2013.

79. Nelson NW, Hoelzle JB, Mcguire KA, et al. Neuropsychological evaluation of blast-related concussion: illustrating the challenges and complexities through OEF/OIF case studies. Brain Inj 2011; 25(5):511–25.

80. Polusny MA, Kehle SM, Nelson NW, et al. Longitudinal effects of mild TBI and PTSD comorbidity on post-deployment outcomes in National Guard soldiers deployed to Iraq. Arch Gen Psychiatry 2011;68:79–89.

81. Vanderploeg RD, Belanger HG, Horner RD, et al. Health outcomes associated with military deployment: mild traumatic brain injury, blast, trauma, and combat associations in the Florida National Guard. Arch Phys Med Rehabil 2012;93(11): 1887–95.

82. Kennedy JE, Cullen MA, Amador RR, et al. Symptoms in military service members after blast mTBI with and without associated injuries. NeuroRehabilitation 2010;26(3):191–7.

83. Uomoto JM, Williams RM, Randa LA. Neurobehavioral consequences of combat-related blast injury and polytrauma. In: Ashley Mark J, editor. Traumatic Brain Injury: Rehabilitation, Treatment, and Case Management, Third Edition. [Online]. CRC Press; 2010. p. 63–95.

84. Carlson KF, Kehle SM, Meis LA, et al. Prevalence, assessment, and treatment of mild traumatic brain injury and posttraumatic stress disorder: a systematic review of the evidence. J Head Trauma Rehabil 2011;26(2):103–15.

85. Pietrzak RH, Johnson DC, Goldstein MB, et al. Posttraumatic stress disorder mediates the relationship between mild traumatic brain injury and health and psychosocial functioning in Veterans of Operations Enduring Freedom and Iraqi Freedom. J Nerv Ment Dis 2009;197(10):748–53.

86. Cohen B, Gima K, Bertenthal D, et al. Mental health diagnoses and utilization of VA non-mental health medical services among returning Iraq and Afghanistan veterans. J Gen Intern Med 2010; 25(1):18–24.

87. Lew HL, Otis JD, Tun C, et al. Prevalence of chronic pain, posttraumatic stress disorder, and persistent postconcussive symptoms in OIF/OEF Veterans: polytrauma clinical triad. J Rehabil Res Dev 2009; 46(6):697–702.

88. Boyle E, Cancelliere C, Hartvigsen J, et al. Systematic review of prognosis after mild traumatic brain injury in the military: results of the International Collaboration on mild traumatic brain injury prognosis. Arch Phys Med Rehabil 2014;95(3 Suppl): S230–7.

89. Luethcke CA, Bryan CJ, Morrow CE, et al. Comparison of concussive symptoms, cognitive performance, and psychological symptoms between acute blast-versus nonblast-induced mild traumatic brain injury. J Int Neuropsychol Soc 2011; 17(1):36–45.

90. Brickell T, Lange R, Bhagwat A, et al. Self-reported symptoms of executive dysfunction and objective neurocognitive performance following military-related Traumatic Brain Injury. Arch Clin Neuropsychol 2013;28(6):606–7.

91. Mortera M, Kinirons S, Simantov J, et al. Patient profile: operation enduring freedom/operation Iraqi Freedom (OEF/OIF) Veterans suspected of traumatic brain injury. Brain Inj 2016;30:5–6. Taylor & Francis Inc.

92. Lange RT, Brickell TA, French LM, et al. Neuropsychological outcome from uncomplicated mild, complicated mild, and moderate traumatic brain injury in US military personnel. Arch Clin Neuropsychol 2012;27(5):480–94.

93. Spencer RJ, Waldron-Perrine B, Drag LL, et al. Neuropsychological test validity in Veterans presenting with subjective complaints of 'very severe' cognitive symptoms following mild traumatic brain injury. Brain Inj 2017;31(1):32–8.

94. Mckee AC, Stern RA, Nowinski CJ, et al. The spectrum of disease in chronic traumatic encephalopathy. Brain 2013;136(Pt 1):43–64.

95. Omalu B, Hammers JL, Bailes J, et al. Chronic traumatic encephalopathy in an Iraqi war veteran with posttraumatic stress disorder who committed suicide. Neurosurg Focus 2011; 31(5):E3.

96. Goldstein LE, Fisher AM, Tagge CA, et al. Chronic traumatic encephalopathy in blast-exposed military Veterans and a blast neurotrauma mouse model. Sci Transl Med 2012;26(4):134ra60.

97. Mckee AC, Cairns NJ, Dickson DW, et al. The first NINDS/NIBIB consensus meeting to define neuropathological criteria for the diagnosis of chronic traumatic encephalopathy. Acta Neuropathol 2016;131(1):75–86.

98. Mckee AC, Robinson ME. Military-related traumatic brain injury and neurodegeneration. Alzheimers Dement 2014;10(3 Suppl):S242–53.

99. High WMJ, Sander AM, Struchen MA, et al. Rehabilitation for traumatic brain injury. New York: Oxford University Press; 2005.

100. Crooks CY, Zumsteg JM, Bell KR. Traumatic brain injury: a review of practice management and recent advances. Phys Med Rehabil Clin N Am 2007; 18(4):681–710, vi.

101. Terrio H, Brenner LA, Ivins BJ, et al. Traumatic brain injury screening: preliminary findings in a US Army Brigade Combat Team. J Head Trauma Rehabil 2009;24(1):14–23.

102. Armistead-Jehle PC, Wesley R, Stegman RL. Performance and symptom validity testing as a function of medical board evaluation in U.S. military service members with a history of mild traumatic brain injury. Arch Clin Neuropsychol 2018;33(1): 120–4.

103. Makdissi M, Cantu RC, Johnston KM, et al. The difficult concussion patient: what is the best approach to investigation and management of persistent (>10 days) postconcussive symptoms? Br J Sports Med 2013;47(5):308–13.

104. Rao V, Syeda A, Roy D, et al. Neuropsychiatric aspects of concussion: acute and chronic sequelae. Concussion 2017;2(1):CNC29.

105. Irimia A, Chambers MC, Alger JR, et al. Comparison of acute and chronic traumatic brain injury using semi-automatic multimodal segmentation of MR volumes. J Neurotrauma 2011;28(11):2287–306.

106. Miller NL, Shattuck LG. Sleep patterns of young men and women enrolled at the United States Military Academy: results from year 1 of a 4-year longitudinal study. Sleep 2005;28(7):837–41.

107. Miller NL, Shattuck LG, Matsangas P. Longitudinal study of sleep patterns of United States Military Academy cadets. Sleep 2010;33(12):1623–31.

108. Mysliwiec V, McGraw L, Pierce R, et al. Sleep disorders and associated medical comorbidities in active duty military personnel. Sleep 2013;36(2): 167–74.

109. Luxton DD, Greenburg D, Ryan J, et al. Prevalence and impact of short sleep duration in redeployed OIF soldiers. Sleep 2011;34(9):1189–95.

110. Harrison E, Glickman G, Rose E, et al. Self-reported sleep during US navy operations and the impact of deployment-related factors. Mil Med 2017;182(3–4):189–94.

111. Capaldi VF, Balkin TJ, Mysliwiec V. Optimizing sleep in the military: challenges and opportunities. Chest 2019;155(1):215–26.

112. Balkin T, Rupp T, Picchioni D, et al. Sleep loss and sleepiness. Chest 2008;134(3):653–63.

113. Belenky G, Wesensten NJ, Thorne DR, et al. Patterns of performance degradation and restoration during sleep restriction and subsequent recovery: a sleep dose-response study. J Sleep Res 2003; 12(1):1–12.

114. Van dongen HP, Maislin G, Mullington JM, et al. The cumulative cost of additional wakefulness: dose-response effects on neurobehavioral functions and sleep physiology from chronic sleep restriction and total sleep deprivation. Sleep 2003;26(2):117–26.

115. Dinges DF, Pack F, Williams K, et al. Cumulative sleepiness, mood disturbance, and psychomotor vigilance performance decrements during a week of sleep restricted to 4-5 hours per night. Sleep 1997;20(4):267–77.

116. Shokri-kojori E, Wang GJ, Wiers CE, et al. β-Amyloid accumulation in the human brain after one night of sleep deprivation. Proc Natl Acad Sci U S A 2018;115(17):4483–8.

117. Van dongen HP, Baynard MD, Maislin G, et al. Systematic interindividual differences in neurobehavioral impairment from sleep loss: evidence of trait-like differential vulnerability. Sleep 2004;27(3): 423–33.

118. Rupp TL, Wesensten NJ, Balkin TJ. Trait-like vulnerability to total and partial sleep loss. Sleep 2012; 35(8):1163–72.

119. Markwald R, Bessman S, Drummond S, et al. Performance during unplanned night time awakenings and following disrupted sleep. J Sci Med Sport 2017;20:S18.

120. Balkin TJ, Badia P. Relationship between sleep inertia and sleepiness: cumulative effects of four nights of sleep disruption/restriction on performance following abrupt nocturnal awakenings. Biol Psychol 1988;27(3):245–58.

121. Scheer FA, Shea TJ, Hilton MF, et al. An endogenous circadian rhythm in sleep inertia results in greatest cognitive impairment upon awakening during the biological night. J Biol Rhythms 2008; 23(4):353–61.

122. Newman RA, Kamimori GH, Wesensten NJ, et al. Caffeine gum minimizes sleep inertia. Percept Mot Skills 2013;116(1):280–93.

123. Lieberman HR, Bathalon GP, Falco CM, et al. Severe decrements in cognition function and mood induced by sleep loss, heat, dehydration, and undernutrition during simulated combat. Biol Psychiatry 2005;57(4):422–9.

124. Rognum TO, Vartdal F, Rodahl K, et al. Physical and mental performance of soldiers on high- and low-energy diets during prolonged heavy exercise combined with sleep deprivation. Ergonomics 1986;29(7):859–67.

125. Belenky G, Penetar DM, Thorne D, et al. The effects of sleep deprivation on performance during continuous combat operations. In: Marriott BM, editor. Food Components to Enhance Performance: An Evaluation of Potential Performance-Enhancing Food Components for Operational Rations. Washington, DC: Institute of Medicine (US) Committee on Military Nutrition Research; 1994. p. 127–36.

126. LoPresti M, Anderson JA, Saboe KN, et al. The impact of insufficient sleep on combat misison performance. Mil Beh Health 2016;4:356–63.

127. Shattuck NL, Matsangas P. Operational assessment of the 5-h on/10-h off watchstanding schedule on a US Navy ship: sleep patterns, mood and psychomotor vigilance performance of crewmembers in the nuclear reactor department. Ergonomics 2016;59(5):657–64.

128. Olsen OK, Pallesen S, Eid J. The impact of partial sleep deprivation on moral reasoning in military officers. Sleep 2010;33(8):1086–90.

129. Hansen AA, Athey AB, Ross MJ, et al. Sleep and health among collegiate student-athletes. Chest 2019;156(6):1234–45.

130. Milewski MD, Skaggs DL, Bishop GA, et al. Chronic lack of sleep is associated with increased sports injuries in adolescent athletes. J Pediatr Orthop 2014;34(2):129–33.

131. Azboy O, Kaygisiz Z. Effects of sleep deprivation on cardiorespiratory functions of the runners and volleyball players during rest and exercise. Acta Physiol Hung 2009;96(1):29–36.

132. Blumert PA, Crum AJ, Ernsting M, et al. The acute effects of twenty-four hours of sleep loss on the performance of national-caliber male collegiate weightlifters. J Strength Cond Res 2007;21(4): 1146–54.

133. Taheri M, Arabameri E. The effect of sleep deprivation on choice reaction time and anaerobic power of college student athletes. Asian J Sports Med 2012;3(1):15–20.

134. Biggins M, Cahalan R, Comyns T, et al. Poor sleep is related to lower general health, increased stress and increased confusion in elite Gaelic athletes. Phys Sportsmed 2018;46(1):14–20.

135. Keramidas ME, Gadefors M, Nilsson LO, et al. Physiological and psychological determinants of whole-body endurance exercise following short-term sustained operations with partial sleep deprivation. Eur J Appl Physiol 2018;118(7):1373–84.

136. Keramidas ME, Siebenmann C, Norrbrand L, et al. A brief pre-exercise nap may alleviate physical performance impairments induced by short-term sustained operations with partial sleep deprivation - a field-based study. Chronobiol Int 2018;35(10): 1464–70.

137. Hsouna H, Boukhris O, Abdessalem R, et al. Effect of different nap opportunity durations on short-term maximal performance, attention, feelings, muscle soreness, fatigue, stress and sleep. Physiol Behav 2019;211:112673.

138. Lucas SJ, Anson JG, Palmer CD, et al. The impact of 100 hours of exercise and sleep deprivation on cognitive function and physical capacities. J Sports Sci 2009;27(7):719–28.

139. Smith CD, Cooper AD, Merullo DJ, et al. Sleep restriction and cognitive load affect performance on a simulated marksmanship task. J Sleep Res 2019;28(3):e12637.

140. Vaara JP, Oksanen H, Kyrolainen H, et al. 60 h sleep deprivation affects submaximal but not maximal physical performance. Front Physiol 2018;9:1437.

141. Nindl B, Leone C, Tharion W, et al. Physical performance responses during 72 h of military operational stress. Med Sci Sports Exerc 2002;34(11):1814–22.

142. Tomczak A, Dabrowski J, Mikulski T. Psychomotor performance of Polish air force cadets after 36 hours survival trainings. Ann Agric Environ Med 2017;24(3):387–91.

143. Tomczak A. Coordination of motor skill of military pilots subjected to survival training. J Strength Cond Res 2015;29(9):2460–4.

144. Lentino CV, Purvis DL, Murphy KJ, et al. Sleep as a component of the performance triad: the importance of sleep in a military population. US Army Med Dep J 2013;98–108.

Brain Stimulation for Improving Sleep and Memory

Roneil G. Malkani, MD, MS[a],*, Phyllis C. Zee, MD, PhD[b]

KEYWORDS

- Slow wave sleep • Memory • Brain stimulation • Acoustic stimulation • Closed-loop stimulation
- Transcranial electric stimulation • Targeted memory reactivation
- Transcranial magnetic stimulation

KEY POINTS

- Transcranial electrical stimulation enhances sleep slow oscillations and can improve declarative memory, but its effects on memory have been inconsistent.
- Transcranial magnetic stimulation during sleep increases slow oscillations, and stimulation during wake improves memory, but the relationship between sleep and memory with this method has not been established.
- Acoustic stimulation in non–rapid eye movement sleep increases slow oscillations, spindles, and their phase coupling, all of which correlate with improvements in declarative memory.
- Targeted memory reactivation in sleep using verbal and nonverbal auditory cues consolidates specific recently encoded memories.
- Future research to determine optimal stimulation parameters and examine long-term safety and effects on cognition and performance is needed in healthy and clinical populations.

INTRODUCTION

Over the past few decades, the importance of sleep has become increasingly recognized for many physiologic functions, including cognition. Many studies have reported the deleterious the effect of sleep loss or sleep disruption on cognitive performance. Beyond ensuring adequate sleep quality and duration, discovering methods to enhance sleep to augment its restorative effects is important to improve learning in many populations, such as the military, students, age-related cognitive decline, and in cognitive disorders. In the past 2 decades, noninvasive sleep stimulation techniques have emerged, including transcranial electrical stimulation, transcranial magnetic stimulation (TMS), acoustic stimulation, and targeted memory reactivation. This article reviews the role of sleep in memory consolidation, these neurostimulation techniques, and their effects on memory.

SLEEP PHYSIOLOGY AND MEMORY
Sleep Physiology

Non–rapid eye movement (NREM) sleep is characterized by cortical neuronal synchrony that increases with deeper stages of NREM sleep. During stage N2 sleep there is a prominence of K-complexes and sleep spindles. Sleep spindles are short bursts of oscillations in the 9-Hz to 15-Hz frequency range that are generated by the thalamic reticular neurons and synchronized by corticothalamic feedback. They are present throughout stage N2 and N3 but are more difficult to visualize during stage N3.[1] Sleep spindles can be divided into slow (10–12 Hz) and fast (13–

[a] Division of Sleep Medicine, Department of Neurology, Center for Circadian and Sleep Medicine, Northwestern University Feinberg School of Medicine. 710 North Lake Shore Drive, Suite 525, Chicago, IL 60611, USA; [b] Division of Sleep Medicine, Department of Neurology, Center for Circadian and Sleep Medicine, Northwestern University Feinberg School of Medicine. 710 North Lake Shore Drive, Suite 520, Chicago, IL 60611, USA
* Corresponding author.
E-mail address: R-malkani@northwestern.edu

Sleep Med Clin 15 (2020) 101–115
https://doi.org/10.1016/j.jsmc.2019.11.002
1556-407X/20/© 2019 Elsevier Inc. All rights reserved.

15 Hz) spindles with differing topographic distribution and functional significance.[2]

The deepest stage of NREM sleep is stage N3, or slow wave sleep (SWS), and is characterized by electroencephalogram (EEG) slow waves in the delta (0.5–4.5 Hz) frequency band. SWS is implicated in many physiologic functions, including cognitive function,[2] hormonal regulation,[1,3,4] immune function, energy saving, and clearance of β-amyloid and toxic metabolites from the brain.[1,5,6] Slow oscillations (SOs), in ~ 1-Hz frequency band, are generated by the thalamocortical system.[7] SOs represent synchronous changes in membrane potential of large populations of cortical neurons in a bistable manner with an upstate and downstate. During the depolarized upstate of the SOs, there is sustained neuronal firing of neurons; during the hyperpolarized downstate, there is neuronal quiescence.[8] SOs originate in the medial prefrontal cortex and propagate posteriorly.[9,10] Stimulation of frontal cortex results in EEG slow waves and sleep,[11] and slow wave activity (SWA; the quantification of power in the delta frequency band using power spectral analysis) is most prominent in the frontal areas.[12]

Rapid eye movement (REM) sleep is characterized by cortical desynchrony, rapid eye movements, and motor atonia that spares respiratory and extraocular muscles. This sleep stage is associated with dreams and seems to play a more important role in procedural and emotional memory.[13,14] Earlier research focused on REM sleep, but recent attention has shifted to SWS. This article focuses on the role of NREM sleep because it has been the target of most of the recent sleep stimulation research.

Learning and Memory

The ability to remember is critical to adapt behaviors in response to the environment. There are 2 general types of memory: declarative and nondeclarative memory. Declarative memory refers to remembering facts and events and relies on the hippocampus. Nondeclarative memory, or procedural memory, refers to unconscious memory of performing a task, such as playing a musical instrument, and depends on corticostriatal and corticocerebellar networks.[2] However, there is some overlap between the memory function of these areas. Memory involves 3 components: encoding, consolidation, and retrieval.[2] During encoding, memory traces are coded and stored in the hippocampus.[15] These memory traces are unstable and are susceptible to interference from other information. Consolidation is the process of stabilization of memories, in which encoded information is

transferred from the hippocampus to the neocortex for long-term storage. This process can occur when awake, but sleep has a critical role in the transfer of memory and integrating information into existing networks.[2,16]

The Role of Sleep in Memory Consolidation

Two major mechanisms have been proposed to explain the role of sleep in memory consolidation: the synaptic homeostasis hypothesis (SHY) and the active system consolidation model. SHY proposes that synaptic strength increases during wake and decreases during sleep, particularly SWS.[17] Because of energy and space constraints, the increase in synaptic density and strength that accumulates while awake is downscaled during sleep.[17] In support of this, markers of synaptic efficacy have been shown to increase while awake and decrease during sleep; these changes are blocked by sleep loss.[18] Furthermore, measures of synaptic strength, such as axon-spine interface, decrease with sleep.[19] Moreover, sleep deprivation increases net synaptic strength and decreases long-term potential-like plasticity.[20] Although SHY explains synaptic downscaling, it does not explain how memories are stored for long-term use or how some memories are retained and others are forgotten.

The active system consolidation model proposes that memories are stored in the hippocampus during encoding while awake. During NREM sleep, memories in the hippocampus are replayed, resulting in transfer of the memory for storage in the neocortex.[21–23] When memories are stabilized in the neocortex, the hippocampus no longer retains the information and returns to a state ready to encode new information.[24] One important unanswered question in this model is how memories are tagged and selected for replay and consolidation.

The SHY and active system consolidation models are not mutually exclusive and may be complementary. These models together could explain how, during sleep, memory replay transfers memories for long-term storage, and synaptic downscaling normalizes synaptic strength, erasing memory traces in the hippocampus, preparing for more learning.

SWS and sleep spindles are of particular importance to the consolidation of declarative memories. Both SWS and spindles[25,26] are independently linked to memory consolidation.[2,27,28] Blocking spindles with electric current impairs memory consolidation.[29] Fast spindles seem to be more consistently linked to memory consolidation, although many studies have not differentiated fast from slow spindles.[2] Sharp wave ripples (SWRs)[30] are 100-Hz to 300-Hz oscillations that originate in the hippocampus and occur in SWS. SWRs increase with learning,[2] and disruption of SWRs impairs memory retention.[29,31]

The current neurophysiologic model of NREM sleep's role in memory consolidation is the interplay between SOs, spindles, and SWRs during SWS. In particular, these waveforms are coordinated in a nested fashion, with spindles occurring during upstate of the SO and SWRs occurring the spindle troughs.[2] This coordination represents the crosstalk between the hippocampus and neocortex that underlies transfer of memories from short-term to long-term storage. This phase coupling seems to occur in a top-down manner with SOs synchronizing thalamocortical spindle and hippocampal SWR generation.[32–35] This phase coupling between SOs, spindles, and SWRs seems to be important for consolidation.[36] Furthermore, increased duration of the SO upstate, which may improve phase locking, is associated with improved declarative memory.[37]

Effect of Aging on Sleep and Memory

Understanding the role of sleep in cognition may be especially important to age-related cognitive decline. After age 55 years, function starts to decline in several cognitive domains, including declarative memory.[38,39] This change parallels reductions in SWS duration.[40] Aging results in decreases in SO density, number, and amplitude and impaired SO propagation.[9,10,41] These changes in SO characteristics may be explained by cortical thinning in areas involved in the default mode network, including medial prefrontal cortex, insula, temporal, and parietal areas.[9] Furthermore, aging decreases the slope and frequency of the SO, indicating decreased neuronal synchrony.[10] There are also reductions in spontaneous K-complexes and sleep spindle number, density, and duration.[42] In addition, aging is associated with reduced phase coupling between SOs and spindles, which predicts poorer overnight memory retention.[33]

Alzheimer's disease (AD) is a neurodegenerative memory disorder associated with aging and that involves deterioration of short-term memory, especially declarative memory. Pathologically, the disease is characterized by extracellular β-amyloid plaques and intracellular tau protein neurofibrillary tangles.[43] As AD progresses, other cognitive domains deteriorate, and patients become unable to independently perform usual activities of daily living. Given that the proportion of elderly is increasing, the prevalence of AD, already at 46.8 million worldwide, is expected to increase to 131.5 million by 2050.[44] Because there is no available cure or disease-modifying therapy, it is imperative to further understand AD and identify risk factors and therapeutic targets for disease prevention and modification. In addition, earlier disease detection may be critical to intervening before significant neurodegeneration.

Sleep disruption has emerged as a potential key player in the pathogenesis of AD. Sleep disturbances are common in people with AD and even confer risk of developing AD.[45] Sleep is involved in regulation of interstitial β-amyloid peptide levels, which increase during wake and decrease during sleep.[46] During sleep deprivation, β-amyloid peptide levels continue to increase while awake; with pharmacologically induced sleep beyond the usual sleep duration, these levels decrease further.[46] This regulation may depend on the glymphatic system, which is responsible for clearance of toxic metabolites from the brain during sleep.[5,6] In addition, reduction in SWS increases levels of tau protein, and sleep fragmentation is associated with the development of tau protein neurofibrillary tangles.[47,48]

Alterations in sleep macrostructure and microstructure can even be seen in people with amnestic mild cognitive impairment (aMCI), a precursor state to AD in which there is memory decline but functional independence is maintained.[49] People with aMCI have lower SWS duration, lower SWA, and lower fast spindle density and count.[28,50] Furthermore, sleep disturbances in people with aMCI are associated with decreased functional connectivity between the prefrontal cortex and temporoparietal junction.[51] Therefore, restoration of normal sleep function is a novel and exciting avenue that may improve cognitive function and even alter the pathophysiology of AD.

METHODS TO ENHANCE SLEEP AND THEIR EFFECTS ON MEMORY

Given the relationship between sleep and memory, there has been growing research in methods to improve memory by modulating sleep. Enhancing sleep for memory has important implications in adults (eg, military, aging, and neurodegenerative disease). Most approaches have targeted SOs and spindles. Enhancing SWS is advantageous because it can occur during daytime naps, making this easier to study and providing more opportunities for therapeutic intervention. The most commonly studied methods include electrical stimulation, magnetic stimulation, acoustic stimulation, and targeted memory reactivation.

Transcranial Electrical Stimulation

Transcranial application of electricity with direct current (DC) or alternating current (AC) can be used to stimulate brain oscillations. Such currents induce neuronal membrane depolarization or hyperpolarization, resulting in entrainment of brain oscillations.[52–54] DC is a unidirectional current that is constant; AC changes in direction, amplitude, frequency, and phase variance/coherence. Transcranial electrical stimulation (TES) can be used to enhance[55] or disrupt[56] oscillations, depending how it is applied. The most common sleep application of TES is for the enhancement of SO, in which case the electrical current is applied at low frequency (typically 0.75 Hz). TES can also be applied at other frequencies (eg, 12 Hz) to stimulate sleep spindles.

Most studies using TES have examined the effects of slow-oscillatory transcranial direct current stimulation (SO-tDCS) on brain oscillations. Marshall and colleagues[57] reported that frontal SO-tDCS applied during a nap in young healthy adults increased frontal SO and delta power. These data led to the landmark study in overnight sleep in healthy young adults that showed enhancement of SO, delta power, and slow sleep spindles.[55] Since then, there have been multiple studies using similar methodology of SO-tDCS during sleep in healthy young and older adults. Most studies show an increase in spectral power in the SO and delta frequency bands during stimulation-free intervals or immediately after stimulation,[55,57–59] although some studies did not.[60–62] Although 1 study showed an increase in SWS,[55] most studies have found no effect on sleep stages, during nap or overnight,[58–60,63,64] and 1 found decreased SWS overnight in older adults.[62]

The effects of tDCS on sleep spindles have been much more varied. Some studies report an increase in fast[63,65] or slow[55] spindle density, whereas others report lower spindle counts[57] or fast spindle density.[64,66] Several other studies with tDCS have found no effect on spindles.[59–62] These discrepancies in spindle effects may be related to several factors, including the type of current, the difference in spindle frequency bands assessed, spindle detection methodologies, and inability to examine the EEG during the stimulation itself.

The effects of TES on cognitive function have also been inconsistent among studies. The initial studies using tDCS showed improvement in word pair association task (WPT), a test of declarative memory that has been used in many studies and is sensitive to sleep effects.[55,57] However, the effect of tDCS on the WPT has been inconsistent,

regardless of how the WPT was given (eg, train to criterion, feedback provided). The mixed results do not seem to depend on the age of population studied or whether the tDCS was applied during a nap or overnight sleep.[60] All studies using tDCS have shown no benefit to procedural memory tasks, consistent with the effect of SWS on declarative memory.[55,57,59–65] One study using transcranial AC stimulation (tACS) showed improvement in a motor sequent tapping task response time but not accuracy.[66]

Although TES has had varied effects in healthy people, there are data to suggest that it may be more effective in clinical populations. For example, because people with aMCI have less SWA, increasing SO may be of particular benefit. One recent study in this population showed that tDCS improved SO power, fast spindle power (12–15 Hz), phase coupling, and visual declarative memory. Furthermore, the memory enhancement correlated with a higher degree of phase coupling.[65] SO-tDCS also improved SO power and memory in children with attention-deficit/hyperactivity disorder[67] and reduced forgetting in adults with paranoid schizophrenia.[68] There are 2 studies using TES in patients with epilepsy. One study using SO-tDCS during wakefulness before a nap in patients with temporal lobe epilepsy found increased total sleep duration, improved declarative verbal memory, and less forgetting of visuospatial memory. Although slow spindle current generator density increased, particularly in frontal areas, fast and slow spindle counts remained unchanged.[69] In contrast, the other study showed that low-frequency tACS during NREM sleep in patients undergoing surgery for medication-refractory epilepsy did not entrain sleep spindles.[70] Each of these populations has had limited data and small sample sizes, and the effects need to be confirmed with additional and larger studies.

Several inherent limitations to TES may explain the discrepancies in these results. First, the dose of current may not be sufficient to stimulate the cortex to reliably increase SWA, because TES affects only the superficial layers of the brain.[57] Second, the parameters of stimulation may need to be individualized to optimize stimulation potential. Third, it remains unclear whether multiple nights of stimulation have lasting and cumulative effects. Fourth, the EEG can be examined only during stimulation-free intervals and after stimulation, not during stimulation, because the application of electrical current interferes with such measurement. In addition, the utility of TES in its present form requires a technician to apply stimulation, limiting at-home or clinical use.

TES is generally safe with no known serious adverse events. Headache, fatigue, tingling, itching, and burning are the most common side effects, with skin lesions occurring under the electrodes in some people with repeated use.[71] However, side effects of nightly long-term use are unknown.

Transcranial Magnetic Stimulation

TMS is a noninvasive neurostimulation technique that can be applied over specific brain areas without requiring physical contact. The magnetic field is generated by passing a strong electric current through a coil positioned over the head by the brain region of interest. The magnetic field stimulates or inhibits nearby neurons and can modulate connected subcortical and transcortical areas.[72] TMS affects cortical neural plasticity, such as long-term potentiation or long-term depression, and can have longer lasting effects than TES, depending on the type and frequency of stimulation. Factors that influence the effects of TMS include the coil shape and orientation, cortical geometry, and TMS type and frequency. TMS can be used as an exploratory tool to assess relationships between brain areas or as a diagnostic tool by assessing functional connectivity as a biomarker. TMS can also be used therapeutically in pain disorders and depression.

TMS can be delivered using different modalities. Single-pulse TMS delivers pulses at least 4 seconds apart to avoid summation of effects. Paired pulse-TMS delivers 2 pulses with varying interstimulation intervals (ISIs) to evaluate conduction times between different brain areas. Repetitive TMS (rTMS) delivers a train of stimuli with ISIs less than 2 seconds apart. rTMS seems to have long-lasting effects and it is the typical modality used therapeutically.[73]

Despite the wealth of data available on TMS effects on the brain, there are sparse data available for its effects on sleep. A few studies have shown that TMS can evoke high-amplitude SO. Massimini and colleagues[74] applied TMS repetitively in blocks of ~0.8 Hz with intertrial intervals of ~1 minute at different midline sites. During NREM sleep, each pulse of the train triggered a high-amplitude SO resembling endogenous SO, which spread to the rest of the brain. The triggered SO upstate was associated with an increase in spindle amplitude. This response was state dependent, because TMS did not evoke SO in the awake state. This effect was also dose and site dependent, with greater stimulation intensity and stimulation over the sensorimotor cortex eliciting the greatest responses.[74] Furthermore, TMS-elicited SOs are larger if the pulse was delivered at the endogenous SO upstate.[75] Single-pulse[76] and paired-pulse TMS[77] techniques also enhanced sleep SO. However, it is unclear whether these induced slow waves serve the same physiologic function as endogenous ones. Further research needs to determine whether increasing trains of SO decrease the need for spontaneous SO, thereby reducing the sleep homeostatic drive, and whether enhancing SO affects cognitive performance.[78]

Although TMS applied in the wake state does not elicit SO, it can increase SWA in subsequent sleep.[79] The increase in SWA was most pronounced where cortical EEG response was most potentiated. This finding was confirmed using a paired associated stimulation protocol, in which the TMS of the motor cortex pulse immediately followed stimulation of the contralateral median nerve. Varying the frequency of stimulation led to either long-term potentiation or depression. If long-term potentiation was seen, SWA was increased in that area during subsequent sleep; if long-term depression was seen, SWA was decreased.[80]

Although studies using TMS have examined either sleep or cognitive effects separately, not linking them together, TMS applied in the wake state improves cognitive performance. For example, rTMS at 5 Hz applied to the midline parietal region improves working memory compared with sham TMS in young adults.[81] Effects are also seen with sleep deprivation, during which rTMS seems to rescue cognitive impairment. Stimulation with rTMS at 5 Hz over the upper occipital region, but not the parietal region, improved working memory after 1 day[82] or 2 days[83] of sleep deprivation. However, rTMS does not improve cognitive performance when given after recovery sleep.[83] One potential mechanism by which TMS improves cognitive function is in facilitating transfer of memories, because it seems to increase functional connectivity between the hippocampus and the stimulated cortical networks.[84]

TMS also has a potential therapeutic role in AD-related cognitive function. Earlier studies showed that rTMS at 20 Hz over the left or right dorsolateral prefrontal cortex improves cognitive function in mild to moderate AD in a single session[85,86] or with repeated sessions over 4 weeks.[87] Combining cognitive training and several sessions of rTMS (20 Hz, 6 stimulation sites, 30 sessions) also improves cognitive function,[88–90] although an optimal control group was not used in these studies. Several small, randomized, sham-controlled trials have also shown benefits in AD (for a review, see Ref.[91]). None of these studies examined the effects of rTMS on sleep EEG, so it is unclear whether sleep effects played a role in the cognitive benefits. Although these studies targeted cortical areas closer to the surface, 1 study used a different coil to stimulate deeper in the brain, specifically the medial prefrontal cortex, and showed improved cognitive performance in a small group of patients with moderate to severe AD.[92] Although this study did not examine effects on sleep, given the role of the medial prefrontal cortex in SWS generation, it is possible that benefits could have been mediated through enhancing sleep.

TMS seems to be safe overall. The most common adverse events reported are headache and fatigue.[93] There are several contraindications to TMS. Ferromagnetic or metallic materials cannot touch the coil. Because seizures have been reported with TMS, although rare, a history of seizures or conditions or medications that lower the seizure threshold are a contraindication. The risk of TMS in pregnancy, heart conditions, and cerebral stimulators is unknown.[73] The major limitations with use of TMS to enhance sleep are related to the interface. TMS requires a trained technician to use. TMS also requires the patient keep the head still, so positioning for stimulation during sleep can be challenging, particularly if considering stimulation throughout the night. Ear plugs and masking sounds need to be used to prevent sleep disruption from the noise from TMS. Furthermore, duration of stimulation is limited because of potential overheating of the coil.[75,78]

Acoustic Stimulation

Another window into the brain to enhance sleep is acoustic stimulation. Sounds provoke a K-complex response, which may be associated with reactive SO.[94] Sound stimuli in sleep activate lemniscal and nonlemniscal pathways through the brainstem to the cortex.[95] The lemniscal pathway projects via the medial geniculate body of the thalamus to the primary auditory cortex. The nonlemniscal pathway projects through 2 parallel pathways to the medial geniculate body and then to the associative cortex. One of the nonlemniscal pathways travels through the locus coeruleus, a wake-promoting nucleus. Activation of the other nonlemniscal pathway results in widespread neuronal depolarization of the cortex. If the sound does not significantly activate the locus coeruleus and result in an arousal, then a K-complex without an arousal results in fast and efficient synchrony and promotes enhancement of the SO.[95] Stimulation does not depend on the side of stimulation, because even unilateral stimulation leads to increased SO in both hemispheres.[96] Nearly all studies on acoustic stimulation have used pink noise (one of the basic types of noise in nature), which comprises a wide range of sound frequencies in a 1/f distribution (ie, lower frequencies provide greater contribution).[97] An advantage of acoustic stimulation is the feasibility and practicality of using an automated system and the ability to develop a device for home use.

Most of the studies using acoustic stimulation have focused on enhancing SO, which is discussed later. However, sleep spindles can also be enhanced with acoustic stimulation. Recently it was shown that oscillating white noise at 12 Hz or 14 Hz can boost slow and fast spindle density, respectively. Although the sounds also increased SO density, the spindle enhancement did not depend on the increase in SO.[98]

There are 2 general types of acoustic stimulation for SO enhancement: open-loop and closed-loop stimulation. Open-loop stimulation consists of delivery of sounds during SWS with the intent to evoke an SO. Sounds are delivered without respect to a particular phase of endogenous SO. Stimulation with trains of 15 to 20 clicks of pink noise at a frequency of 0.8 to 2 Hz during NREM sleep increased SWA throughout the night.[99] One recent study with open-loop low-frequency stimulation with 3 tones in a sequence also increased SO but decreased fast and slow spindle power and did not improve declarative memory.[100]

In contrast with open loop stimulation, closed-loop stimulation bases the timing of the sequence of tones to a targeted phase of endogenous SO to enhance them. This methodology involves monitoring the EEG in real time to identify SOs in SWS and deliver the sounds on a specific phase of the SO. Most recent studies of acoustic stimulation using a form of closed-loop stimulation are based on the seminal work from and Ngo and colleagues[101] in young adults. In this study, an algorithm for online detection of SO identified the negative half-wave of the SO and then delivered 2 clicks of pink noise. The first click occurred about 0.5 seconds after the negative peak of the SO to target the SO upstate. This delay was based on the interval between the negative peak and positive peak measured on the adaptation night. The second click occurred a fixed interval of 1.075 seconds after the first. This method enhanced the amplitude of SO and fast and slow spindle power without increasing overall SWA across the night or changing sleep stage duration or distribution. The increase in SO power occurred predominantly in the frontal leads, much like the natural topographic distribution of SO power in humans. Furthermore, stimulation increased performance on the declarative memory task (WPT);

this improvement correlated with increase in fast spindle power.

Timing of stimuli seems to matter to some extent, although train length may not. Delivery of the sounds during the negative peak of the SO enhanced neither SWA nor memory.[101] Randomly timed stimulation did not increase SO power but increased fast spindle power.[102] Because 2-click stimulation increased SWA, it was plausible that increasing train length of stimuli would increase SWA further. However, stimulating continuously in the presence of SO to drive SO did not improve SWA any better that the 2-click paradigm.[103]

Similar protocols assessing 1-tone or 2-tone trains of stimulation also enhanced SWA.[104–106] A 1-tone stimulation method increased SWA and spindle power and improved declarative memory with WPT but not procedural memory.[104] This study also found that spindle activity increased at the peak of SO.[104]

An interesting point about acoustic stimulation of SO is that it seems to alter brain oscillations during stimulation but preserves the overall sleep architecture and spectral power. Most studies found no significant change in sleep stage duration or proportion[101–105,107–110] or in overall SWA.[101,108,109,111] Only 1 showed increase in SWA in young adults.[107] With the phase-locked loop (PLL) method, there is an increase in SO power during trains of stimulation but a decrease between trains, suggesting a reorganization of SO. The changes between the trains of stimulation and the intertrain intervals were particularly associated with change in declarative memory performance[108,109] and autonomic function,[111] indicating that the reorganization of SO may be critical for memory consolidation.

Another emerging form of closed-loop stimulation is PLL stimulation. This method uses an automated algorithm that phase locks to the EEG and track SO in real time with the intent of delivering the sounds at the SO upstate (**Fig. 1**).[109,112] The potential advantage is that delivery of the sounds after the first tone in the block is most likely to be at the upstate. Other forms of closed-loop stimulation delivered the sound a fixed interval after the initial tone of the train, but delivery of subsequent tones on the upstate may be not precise because the frequency of SO can vary. The PLL phase targeting is precise[108–110,112] and the PLL method enhances SO and increases fast spindle activity in young adults during a nap.[110] In older adults, it increases SO power and spindle density and amplitude during overnight sleep (**Fig. 2**)[109] and is associated with better performance on the WPT.

Acoustic stimulation may also have effects beyond memory. In particular, stimulation seems to affect immune function,[105] reduce cortisol levels,[105,111] increase parasympathetic tone during sleep, and decrease sympathetic tone in the morning after stimulation.[111]

The ability of acoustic stimulation to enhance SWA persists even after multiple nights of stimulation. A recent study used a commercially available acoustic stimulation device for at-home use.[106] The validation study showed an increase in SO amplitude using a 2-tone PLL method to deliver pink noise via bone conduction through the mastoid in healthy young adults. SO amplitude enhancement was similar on the first and the tenth consecutive night of stimulation. Therefore, the brain does not seem to adapt to stimulation in a way that would limit long-term effects on SO.[106] Another protocol assessing stimulation of multiple nights used a different portable system that has an automated detection system to deliver a tone to the SO upstate followed by stimulation at 1-second intervals during NREM sleep.[107] Over a 5-night period, compared with sham, patients younger than 40 years had SWA enhancement even after the fifth night of stimulation; however, those more than 40 years old did not have SWA enhancement. The lack of effect seen in those more than 40 years old may be influenced by sensitivity of SWS detection, which was much lower in this group compared with the younger group, or the method of stimulation,[107] because the PLL method did enhance SWA in older adults.[109] Neither study with multiple nights of stimulation examined the effects of acoustic stimulation on memory.

Many of these studies assessed stimulation in young adults. Given that SWA declines with aging,[40,41] and that reductions in SWA relate to declarative memory performance in older adults,[28,41] SWA enhancement in middle-aged and older adults may be a feasible way to mitigate age-related decline in declarative memory. Only 2 studies have examined acoustic stimulation in middle-aged people. In 1 study, acoustic stimulation enhanced SO amplitude in young to middle-aged people (mean age, 40.8 years). The longitudinal analysis showed enhancement after 10 nights in those with mean age 45.4 years[106] but did not separately report young versus middle-aged adults. In contrast, another study showed no enhancement in those more than 40 years of age.[107] These differences may be caused by differences in either SO detection or sound delivery methods. However, the PLL method with trains of 5 clicks with a refractory period of about 5 to 6 seconds showed enhancement of SWA and fast spindle power and improvement in WPT performance in older adults.[109]

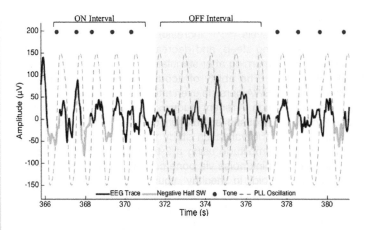

Fig. 1. A sample of electroencephalographic data (*solid black line*) with concurrent PLL acoustic stimulation. The PLL (*dashed gray line*) oscillates with variable frequency to match the endogenous slow oscillations. During trains of stimulation (ON intervals), the tone of pink noise (*red dots*) is played just before the peak of the positive upstate for 5 PLL oscillations. During periods between trains (OFF intervals), no tones are given for 5 PLL oscillations. (*Adapted from* Papalambros NA, Santostasi G, Malkani RG, et al. Acoustic Enhancement of Sleep Slow Oscillations and Concomitant Memory Improvement in Older Adults. *Front Hum Neurosci.* 2017;11(March):1-14; with permission.)

Therefore, acoustic stimulation has potential to improve sleep quality and memory in older adults.

Because people with aMCI have reduced SWA,[28] enhancing SO with acoustic stimulation may be a feasible method to mitigate cognitive dysfunction in aMCI. The PLL method of acoustic stimulation enhances SO in people with aMCI.[108] The degree of enhancement correlates with improvement in WPT performance, showing that even people with cognitive impairment retain adequate brain plasticity and integrity such that SO enhancement can improve memory. However, this effect was examined in a small sample and over only 1 night of stimulation, and it is unclear whether these potential benefits will be seen after multiple nights of stimulation.[108]

Although acoustic stimulation enhances SWA and sleep-sensitive declarative memory performance, there are several unanswered questions on optimal stimulation parameters.[95] First, the optimal timing of stimulation needs to be determined. Stimulation of the downstate of the SO does not seem to enhance SO.[101] However, it is unclear how precisely and accurately the sound stimulus needs to be delivered at the upstate of the SO to best enhance SWA. Because the closed-loop and PLL systems deliver sounds differently, one system may be more effective than the other at enhancing SWA, but this remains to be determined. Second, the optimal sound to enhance SWA is unclear. Most studies used pink noise in 50-millisecond pulses. Some used a ramping on and off with the pulse, whereas others did not. Other pulse durations or frequency distributions may also be effective, but studies are lacking. Third, the optimal volume for stimulation needs to be determined. Some studies have used a fixed volume, whereas others used an

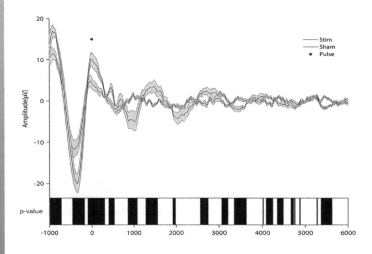

Fig. 2. A grand average event-related potential using PLL acoustic stimulation in older adults. The EEG of trains of stimulation (ON intervals with stimulation [Stim]) and trains of sham stimulation (ON intervals with sham) are aligned to the first tone (*purple dot*). In the sham condition, the timing of tone delivery is marked but no tones are given. Stimulation (*red line*) results in increased slow oscillation amplitude compared with sham (*blue line*). Because frequency of the PLL varies within each train, the remaining tones of each train are not shown. The black bars below indicate statistical significance (*P*<.05) between conditions. (*Adapted from* Papalambros NA, Santostasi G, Malkani RG, et al. Acoustic Enhancement of Sleep Slow Oscillations and Concomitant Memory Improvement in Older Adults. *Front Hum Neurosci.* 2017;11(March):1-14; with permission.)

adaptive volume to deliver sounds, but it is unclear whether one method is more effective that the other and what the optimal volume adjustment method is. Fourth, entrainment of SOs may vary based on number of stimuli delivered in a train of SOs. Although 1 study did not show any benefit with continuous stimulation,[103] another showed that cumulative SWA increased with continuous stimulation.[107] However, continuous stimulation may lead to habituation, so intermittent stimulation across the night, as most studies have done with short trains of stimuli, may be more effective. In addition, different populations may need different parameters. For example, older adults may need different sleep stage and SO detection parameters to start stimulation and may need different timing, sound, volume, or train length to optimally improve SWA.

Acoustic stimulation has some limitations. First, only sleep-sensitive tasks such as the WPT have shown improvements. Effects on other tasks of declarative memory and long-term effects have yet to be shown. Second, long-term effects on cognitive performance have not yet been shown, and it is unclear whether repeated sessions will continue to benefit cognition. No adverse events from acoustic stimulation have yet been reported.

Targeted Memory Reactivation

Both TES and acoustic stimulation enhance SWA and perhaps spindles to nonspecifically enhance declarative memory, but recent strategies have emerged to enhance specific memories. Because recently encoded memories are replayed during sleep-mediated consolidation, it may be possible to selectively replay specific memories to enhance their consolidation. Targeted memory reactivation (TMR) uses a sensory cue paired with information during encoding, and the cue is replayed during sleep to reactivate the associated memory and promote its consolidation.

Reactivation using cues is hippocampal dependent. Replaying during sleep an odor cue associated with recently encoded information increases hippocampal activity during sleep[113] and improves hippocampal-dependent declarative memories but not hippocampal-independent procedural memories.[113] Furthermore, people with greater hippocampal volume have greater response to TMR, and people with bilateral hippocampal sclerosis do not respond to TMR.[114]

Several types of cues have been used (odor, nonverbal auditory, and verbal cues) and can improve memory. Odor cues are less likely to cause an arousal during sleep than an auditory cue, and TMR with odor cues can strengthen hippocampal-dependent memory.[113]

Several studies have used nonverbal cues to reactivate and strengthen memories.[115–118] Replaying a melody during a nap enhances the recall and performance of playing that melody correctly.[119] This enhancement is accomplished by pairing a sound with information to be encoded. These studies then replay half of the sounds and examine which memories were better consolidated. Most studies tested memory with the picture-location task, a test of declarative memory, in which the patient learns the location of various objects (eg, cat) while a sound is played (eg, a meow). On the recall test, the patient reports the location of the presented object.[116–118,120,121] TMR reduces forgetting of cued items across several studies when done during a nap or overnight sleep.[116–118,120] TMR with nonverbal sounds can also alter proprioceptive and body ownership memory as tested using a rubber hand.[122]

TMR using verbal cues also reduces forgetting on the WPT.[121] This finding does not seem to be caused only by the sound but also by the word. Changing the verbal cue from a male to female voice alters the sound but not the meaning of the word cue. This change effectively reduced forgetting in cued and noncued memories. These data indicate that word memories are stored in an episodic form (with speaker detail) and abstract, speaker-independent form.[121,123]

TMR can also rescue memories that may have been forgotten. When value or importance is given to information during encoding, higher value information is consolidated more effectively. When sounds associated with object location of low-value items are played, low-value memories are also consolidated similarly to high-value memories.

Emotional memory may also be altered by TMR. Groch and colleagues[124] tested healthy adolescents and young adults on positive and negative memories. Subjects were shown ambiguous pictures and then either a positive or negative word, and half the positive and negative words were replayed in sleep. Not only was recall better for cued items but cueing with positive words led to more positive interpretations, and cueing negative words led to less positive interpretations of new pictures.[124]

Recent data have shown that the timing of TMR may be important to improve memory. The time of TMR relative to encoding has different effects on memory. If TMR is done soon after encoding, TMR with sounds improves object location memory. However, if TMR is delayed (hours later), then TMR weakens the memory.[117] In addition, the timing relative to the phase of SO may be critical. When cues were delivered between the peak of the upstate and the trough of the downstate of the SO, TMR led to less forgetting than if the cue was delivered in the other phase half.[118] The difference in timing relative to what has been tested in acoustic stimulation may be caused by the time needed to reach the auditory cortex and additional auditory processing needed to reactivate memories.[118]

There are several unanswered questions regarding the use of TMR.[115] First, the underlying neural mechanisms still need to be elucidated, including how cues activate certain memories and which neural pathways are involved. Second, the fidelity of the memory replayed is also unclear, including whether replayed memories are always exact or some memories are distorted. It is also unclear whether memories can be distorted. Third, the effects of repeated TMR are also unknown, including whether the effects are cumulative and enduring and whether the effects are generalizable across the lifespan. Fourth, TMR has potential to be used therapeutically, and clinical application needs to be tested. TMR has specific advantages compared with other techniques because of its targeted nature. For example, given the effects on positive and negative bias, TMR can potentially address unpleasant memories in people with posttraumatic stress disorder or help treat undesired habits. Answers to these important questions will be critical to better understand the role of memory replay in sleep and to develop clinical tools to enhance memory.

TMR also has several inherent limitations. First, TMR requires a learning program with built-in cues, and learned information is likely specific to that learning program. Second, there are limits to the number of cues that can be replayed during the finite amount of SWS. Third, although TMR improves cued memories, this enhancement may be at the expense of uncued memories, indicating a consolidation bias.[125] Although there are no known adverse events from TMR, further data are needed to confirm the tolerability of TMR.

SUMMARY

Sleep's role in memory consolidation represents a critical avenue to improve the quality and effectiveness of sleep and memory. Multiple techniques have emerged to enhance sleep to improve declarative memory. Although TES increases SOs between stimulation periods or after stimulation, the effects on spindles and on memory are inconsistent in healthy people. Furthermore, the utility of TES is limited because it requires a trained technician to apply the electrodes. TMS can elicit and enhance SWA locally and globally and improves cognitive function, but it is unclear whether its effects on memory are linked to sleep. Although the TMS interface limits its potential therapeutic utility to enhance SO during sleep, stimulation when awake may have potential benefits on sleep-related memory consolidation, but this requires further examination. Acoustic stimulation during sleep has been shown to enhance SOs and spindle activity and the phase relationship between the two. Furthermore, acoustic stimulation more consistently improves declarative memory and seems to have benefits in clinical populations. A significant advantage of acoustic stimulation is that it is easily adaptable for home use, and devices for auditory stimulation are already developed. TMR enhances selected information using associated cues and has particular relevance when specific information needs to be consolidated preferentially. A unique feature of TMR is that, in addition to improving declarative memory, it may also rescue forgotten memories with the potential to alter emotional memories. Several unanswered questions need to be addressed for each of these techniques, including safety, long-term effects, and optimal parameters for a given person and therapeutic utility. Future development of neurostimulation systems for therapeutic applications is promising for age-related cognitive disorders as well as sleep disorders.

DISCLOSURE

R.G. Malkani has nothing to disclose. Dr P.C. Zee is an inventor on a patent application for the PLL technique of acoustic stimulation that has been filed by Northwestern University with the United States Patent and Trademark Office (US Patent Application Number 15/517,458). Dr P.C. Zee also serves on the Philips scientific advisory board.

ACKNOWLEDGMENTS

This manuscript was supported in part by the Northwestern University Feinberg School of Medicine Center for Circadian and Sleep Medicine.

REFERENCES

1. Léger D, Debellemaniere E, Rabat A, et al. Slow-wave sleep: from the cell to the clinic. Sleep Med Rev 2018;41:113–32.
2. Rasch B, Born J. About sleep's role in memory. Physiol Rev 2013;93(2):681–766.
3. Tasali E, Leproult R, Ehrmann DA, et al. Slow-wave sleep and the risk of type 2 diabetes in humans. Proc Natl Acad Sci U S A 2008;105(3):1044–9.

4. Van Cauter E, Spiegel K, Tasali E, et al. Metabolic consequences of sleep and sleep loss. Sleep Med 2008;9(suppl 1):S23–8.

5. Xie L, Kang H, Xu Q, et al. Sleep drives metabolite clearance from the adult brain. Science 2013; 342(6156):373–7.

6. Roh JH, Huang Y, Bero AW, et al. Disruption of the sleep-wake cycle and diurnal fluctuation of amyloid-β in mice with Alzheimer's disease pathology. Sci Transl Med 2012;4(150):150ra122.

7. Amzica F, Steriade M. Cellular substrates and laminar profile of sleep K-complex. Neuroscience 1997;82(3):671–86.

8. Amzica F, Steriade M. Electrophysiological correlates of sleep delta waves. Electroencephalogr Clin Neurophysiol 1998;107:69–83.

9. Dubè J, Lafortune M, Bedetti C, et al. Cortical thinning explains changes in sleep slow waves during adulthood. J Neurosci 2015;35(20):7795–807.

10. Carrier J, Viens I, Poirier G, et al. Sleep slow wave changes during the middle years of life. Eur J Neurosci 2011;33(4):758–66.

11. Sterman MB, Clemente CD. Forebrain inhibitory mechanisms: sleep patterns induced by basal forebrain stimulation in the behaving cat. Exp Neurol 1962;6(2):103–17.

12. Massimini M, Huber R, Ferrarelli F, et al. The sleep slow oscillation as a traveling wave. J Neurosci 2004;24(31):6862–70.

13. Plihal W, Born J. Effects of early and late nocturnal sleep on declarative and procedural memory. J Cogn Neurosci 1997;9(4):534–47.

14. Groch S, Zinke K, Wilhelm I, et al. Dissociating the contributions of slow-wave sleep and rapid eye movement sleep to emotional item and source memory. Neurobiol Learn Mem 2015;122: 122–30.

15. Frankland PW, Bontempi B. The organization of recent and remote memories. Nat Rev Neurosci 2005;6(2):119–30.

16. Sutherland GR, McNaughton B. Memory trace reactivation in hippocampal and neocortical neuronal ensembles. Curr Opin Neurobiol 2000;10(2):180–6.

17. Tononi G, Cirelli C. Sleep and the price of plasticity: from synaptic and cellular homeostasis to memory consolidation and integration. Neuron 2014;81(1): 12–34.

18. Cirelli C. Sleep, synaptic homeostasis and neuronal firing rates. Curr Opin Neurobiol 2017;44:72–9.

19. De Vivo L, Bellesi M, Marshall W, et al. Ultrastructural evidence for synaptic scaling across the wake/sleep cycle. Science 2017;355(6324):507–10.

20. Kuhn M, Wolf E, Maier JG, et al. Sleep recalibrates homeostatic and associative synaptic plasticity in the human cortex. Nat Commun 2016;7:12455.

21. Born J, Wilhelm I. System consolidation of memory during sleep. Psychol Res 2012;76(2):192–203.

22. Diekelmann S, Born J. The memory function of sleep. Nat Rev Neurosci 2010;11(2):114–26.

23. Buzsáki G. Memory consolidation during sleep: a neurophysiological perspective. J Sleep Res 1998;7(S1):17–23.

24. Van Der Werf YD, Altena E, Schoonheim MM, et al. Sleep benefits subsequent hippocampal functioning. Nat Neurosci 2009;12(2):122–3.

25. Gais S, Mölle M, Helms K, et al. Learning-dependent increases in sleep spindle density. J Neurosci 2002;22(15):6830–4.

26. Schabus M, Gruber G, Parapatics S, et al. Sleep spindles and their significance for declarative memory consolidation. Sleep 2004;27(8): 1479–85.

27. Chauvette S, Seigneur J, Timofeev I. Sleep oscillations in the thalamocortical system induce long-term neuronal plasticity. Neuron 2012;75(6): 1105–13.

28. Westerberg CE, Mander BA, Florczak SM, et al. Concurrent impairments in sleep and memory in amnestic mild cognitive impairment. J Int Neuropsychol Soc 2012;18(3):490–500.

29. Girardeau G, Benchenane K, Wiener SI, et al. Selective suppression of hippocampal ripples impairs spatial memory. Nat Neurosci 2009;12(10):1222–3.

30. Buzsáki G, Horváth Z, Urioste R, et al. High-frequency network oscillation in the hippocampus. Science 1992;256(5059):1025–7.

31. Ego-Stengel V, Wilson MA. Disruption of ripple-associated hippocampal activity during rest impairs spatial learning in the rat. Hippocampus 2010;20(1):1–10.

32. Klinzing JG, Mölle M, Weber F, et al. Spindle activity phase-locked to sleep slow oscillations. Neuroimage 2016;134:607–16.

33. Helfrich RF, Mander BA, Jagust WJ, et al. Old brains come uncoupled in sleep: slow wave-spindle synchrony, brain atrophy, and forgetting. Neuron 2018;97(1):221–30.

34. Steriade M, McCormick DA, Sejnowski TJ. Thalamocortical oscillations in the sleeping and aroused brain. Science 1993;262(5134):679–85.

35. Steriade M, Contreras D, Amzica F. Synchronized sleep oscillations and their paroxysmal developments. Trends Neurosci 1994;17(5):199–208.

36. Maingret N, Girardeau G, Todorova R, et al. Hippocampo-cortical coupling mediates memory consolidation during sleep. Nat Neurosci 2016;19(7): 959–64.

37. Heib DPJ, Hoedlmoser K, Anderer P, et al. Slow oscillation amplitudes and up-state lengths relate to memory improvement. PLoS One 2013;8(12): e82049.

38. Hedden T, Gabrieli JDE. Insights into the ageing mind: a view from cognitive neuroscience. Nat Rev Neurosci 2004;5(2):87–96.

39. Schaie KW. Intellectual development in adulthood: the Seattle longitudinal study. Cambridge (England): Cambridge University Press; 1996.

40. Ohayon MM, Carskadon MA, Guilleminault C, et al. Meta-analysis of quantitative sleep parameters from childhood to old age in healthy individuals: developing normative sleep values across the human lifespan. Sleep 2004;27(7):1255–73.

41. Mander BA, Rao V, Lu B, et al. Prefrontal atrophy, disrupted NREM slow waves and impaired hippocampal-dependent memory in aging. Nat Neurosci 2013;16(3):357–64.

42. Crowley K, Trinder J, Kim Y, et al. The effects of normal aging on sleep spindle and K-complex production. Clin Neurophysiol 2002;113(10):1615–22.

43. Masters CL, Simms G, Weinman NA, et al. Amyloid plaque core protein in Alzheimer disease and Down syndrome. Proc Natl Acad Sci U S A 1985; 82:4245–9.

44. Prince M, Wimo A, Guerchet M, et al. World Alzheimer Report 2015: the global impact of dementia: an analysis, of prevalence, incidence, cost, and trends. London: Alzheimer's Disease International; 2015.

45. Shi L, Chen S-J, Ma M-Y, et al. Sleep disturbances increase the risk of dementia: a systematic review and meta-analysis. Sleep Med Rev 2017. https://doi.org/10.1016/j.smrv.2017.06.010.

46. Kang J-E, Lim MM, Bateman RJ, et al. Amyloid-beta dynamics are regulated by orexin and the sleep-wake cycle. Science 2009;326(5955):1005–7.

47. Liguori C, Romigi A, Nuccetelli M, et al. Orexinergic system dysregulation, sleep impairment, and cognitive decline in Alzheimer disease. JAMA Neurol 2014;71(12):1498–505.

48. Lim ASP, Yu L, Kowgier M, et al. Modification of the relationship of the apolipoprotein E ε4 allele to the risk of Alzheimer disease and neurofibrillary tangle density by sleep. JAMA Neurol 2013;70(12):1544–51.

49. Petersen RC. Mild cognitive impairment as a clinical entity. J Intern Med 2004;256(7):183–94.

50. Gorgoni M, Lauri G, Truglia I, et al. Parietal fast sleep spindle density decrease in Alzheimer's disease and amnesic mild cognitive impairment. Neural Plast 2016;2016:8376108.

51. McKinnon AC, Duffy SL, Cross NE, et al. Functional connectivity in the default mode network is reduced in association with nocturnal awakening in mild cognitive impairment. J Alzheimers Dis 2017;56(4):1373–84.

52. Herrmann CS, Rach S, Neuling T, et al. Transcranial alternating current stimulation: a review of the underlying mechanisms and modulation of cognitive processes. Front Hum Neurosci 2013; 7:279.

53. Antal A, Herrmann CS. Transcranial alternating current and random noise stimulation: possible mechanisms. Neural Plast 2016;3616807. https://doi.org/10.1155/2016/3616807.

54. Jackson MP, Rahman A, Lafon B, et al. Animal models of transcranial direct current stimulation: methods and mechanisms. Clin Neurophysiol 2016;127(11):3425–54.

55. Marshall L, Helgadóttir H, Mölle M, et al. Boosting slow oscillations during sleep potentiates memory. Nature 2006;444(7119):610–3.

56. Garside P, Arizpe J, Lau CI, et al. Cross-hemispheric alternating current stimulation during a nap disrupts slow wave activity and associated memory consolidation. Brain Stimul 2015;8(3):520–7.

57. Marshall L, Mölle M, Hallschmid M, et al. Transcranial direct current stimulation during sleep improves declarative memory. J Neurosci 2004; 24(44):9985–92.

58. Ladenbauer J, Külzow N, Passmann S, et al. Brain stimulation during an afternoon nap boosts slow oscillatory activity and memory consolidation in older adults. Neuroimage 2016;142:311–23.

59. Paßmann S, Külzow N, Ladenbauer J, et al. Boosting slow oscillatory activity using tDCS during early nocturnal slow wave sleep does not improve memory consolidation in healthy older adults. Brain Stimul 2016;9(5):730–9.

60. Bueno-Lopez A, Eggert T, Dorn H, et al. Slow oscillatory transcranial direct current stimulation (so-tDCS) during slow wave sleep has no effects on declarative memory in healthy young subjects. Brain Stimul 2019;12(4):948–58.

61. Sahlem GL, Badran BW, Halford JJ, et al. Oscillating square wave transcranial direct current stimulation (tDCS) delivered during slow wave sleep does not improve declarative memory more than sham: a randomized sham controlled crossover study. Brain Stimul 2015;8(3):528–34.

62. Eggert T, Dorn H, Sauter C, et al. No effects of slow oscillatory transcranial direct current stimulation (tDCS) on sleep-dependent memory consolidation in healthy elderly subjects. Brain Stimul 2013;6:938–45.

63. Koo PC, Mölle M, Marshall L. Efficacy of slow oscillatory-transcranial direct current stimulation on EEG and memory – contribution of an inter-individual factor. Eur J Neurosci 2018;47(7):812–23.

64. Westerberg CE, Florczak SM, Weintraub S, et al. Memory improvement via slow-oscillatory stimulation during sleep in older adults. Neurobiol Aging 2015;36(9):2577–86.

65. Ladenbauer J, Ladenbauer J, Külzow N, et al. Promoting sleep oscillations and their functional coupling by transcranial stimulation enhances

memory consolidation in mild cognitive impairment. J Neurosci 2017;37(30):7111–24.

66. Lustenberger C, Boyle MR, Alagapan S, et al. Feedback-controlled transcranial alternating current stimulation reveals a functional role of sleep spindles in motor memory consolidation. Curr Biol 2016;26(16):2127–36.

67. Prehn-Kristensen A, Munz M, Göder R, et al. Transcranial oscillatory direct current stimulation during sleep improves declarative memory consolidation in children with attention-deficit/hyperactivity disorder to a level comparable to healthy controls. Brain Stimul 2014;7(6):793–9.

68. Göder R, Baier PC, Beith B, et al. Effects of transcranial direct current stimulation during sleep on memory performance in patients with schizophrenia. Schizophr Res 2013;144:153–4.

69. Del Felice A, Magalini A, Masiero S. Slow-oscillatory transcranial direct current stimulation modulates memory in temporal lobe epilepsy by altering sleep spindle generators: a possible rehabilitation tool. Brain Stimul 2015;8(3):567–73.

70. Lafon B, Henin S, Huang Y, et al. Low frequency transcranial electrical stimulation does not entrain sleep rhythms measured by human intracranial recordings. Nat Commun 2017;8(1):1199.

71. Antal A, Alekseichuk I, Bikson M, et al. Low intensity transcranial electric stimulation: safety, ethical, legal regulatory and application guidelines. Clin Neurophysiol 2017;128(9):1774–809.

72. Luber B, McClintock SM, Lisanby SH. Applications of transcranial magnetic stimulation and magnetic seizure therapy in the study and treatment of disorders related to cerebral aging. Dialogues Clin Neurosci 2013;15:87–98.

73. Babiloni AH, De Beaumont L, Lavigne GJ. Transcranial magnetic stimulation: potential use in obstructive sleep apnea and sleep bruxism. Sleep Med Clin 2018;13(4):571–82.

74. Massimini M, Ferrarelli F, Esser SK, et al. Triggering sleep slow waves by transcranial magnetic stimulation. Proc Natl Acad Sci U S A 2007;104(20): 8496–501.

75. Bergmann TO, Mölle M, Schmidt MA, et al. EEG-guided transcranial magnetic stimulation reveals rapid shifts in motor cortical excitability during the human sleep slow oscillation. J Neurosci 2012; 32(1):243–53.

76. Manganotti P, Formaggio E, Del Felice A, et al. Time-frequency analysis of short-lasting modulation of EEG induced by TMS during wake, sleep deprivation and sleep. Front Hum Neurosci 2013; 7:767.

77. Stamm M, Aru J, Rutiku R, et al. Occipital long-interval paired pulse TMS leads to slow wave components in NREM sleep. Conscious Cogn 2015;35: 78–87.

78. Massimini M, Tononi G, Huber R. Slow waves, synaptic plasticity and information processing: insights from transcranial magnetic stimulation and high-density EEG experiments. Eur J Neurosci 2009;29(9):1761–70.

79. Huber R, Esser SK, Ferrarelli F, et al. TMS-induced cortical potentiation during wakefulness locally increases slow wave activity during sleep. PLoS One 2007;2(3):e276.

80. Huber R, Määttä S, Esser SK, et al. Measures of cortical plasticity after transcranial paired associative stimulation predict changes in electroencephalogram slow-wave activity during subsequent sleep. J Neurosci 2008;28(31):7911–8.

81. Luber B, Kinnunen LH, Rakitin BC, et al. Facilitation of performance in a working memory task with rTMS stimulation of the precuneus: frequency- and time-dependent effects. Brain Res 2007; 1128(1):120–9.

82. Martinez-Cancino DP, Azpiroz-Leehan J, Jimenez-Angeles L, et al. Effects of high frequency rTMS on sleep deprivation: a pilot study. Conf Proc IEEE Eng Med Biol Soc 2016;2016:5937–40.

83. Luber B, Stanford AD, Bulow P, et al. Remediation of sleep-deprivation-induced working memory impairment with fMRI-guided transcranial magnetic stimulation. Cereb Cortex 2008;18:2077–85.

84. Wang JX, Rogers LM, Gross EZ, et al. Memory enhancement: targeted enhancement of cortical-hippocampal brain networks and associative memory. Science 2014;345(6200):1054–7.

85. Cotelli M, Manenti R, Cappa SF, et al. Effect of transcranial magnetic stimulation on action naming in patients with Alzheimer disease. Arch Neurol 2006;63(11):1602–4.

86. Cotelli M, Manenti R, Cappa SF, et al. Transcranial magnetic stimulation improves naming in Alzheimer disease patients at different stages of cognitive decline. Eur J Neurol 2008;15(12): 1286–92.

87. Cotelli M, Calabria M, Manenti R, et al. Improved language performance in Alzheimer disease following brain stimulation. J Neurol Neurosurg Psychiatry 2011;82(7):794–7.

88. Bentwich J, Dobronevsky E, Aichenbaum S, et al. Beneficial effect of repetitive transcranial magnetic stimulation combined with cognitive training for the treatment of Alzheimer's disease: a proof of concept study. J Neural Transm 2011;118(3): 463–71.

89. Rabey JM, Dobronevsky E. Repetitive transcranial magnetic stimulation (rTMS) combined with cognitive training is a safe and effective modality for the treatment of Alzheimer's disease: clinical experience. J Neural Transm 2016;123(12):1449–55.

90. Lee J, Choi BH, Oh E, et al. Treatment of Alzheimer's disease with repetitive transcranial

magnetic stimulation combined with cognitive training: a prospective, randomized, double-blind, placebo-controlled study. J Clin Neurol 2016; 12(1):57–64.

91. Buss SS, Fried PJ, Pascual-Leone A. Therapeutic noninvasive brain stimulation in Alzheimer's disease and related dementias. Curr Opin Neurol 2019;32(2):292–304.

92. Avirame K, Stehberg J, Todder D. Benefits of deep transcranial magnetic stimulation in Alzheimer disease case series. J ECT 2016;32(2): 127–33.

93. Chang C-H, Lane H-Y, Lin C-H. Brain stimulation in Alzheimer's disease. Front Psychiatry 2018;9:201.

94. Halász P. The K-complex as a special reactive sleep slow wave - A theoretical update. Sleep Med Rev 2016;29:34–40.

95. Bellesi M, Riedner BA, Garcia-Molina GN, et al. Enhancement of sleep slow waves: underlying mechanisms and practical consequences. Front Syst Neurosci 2014;8:208.

96. Simor P, Steinbach E, Nagy T, et al. Lateralized rhythmic acoustic stimulation during daytime NREM sleep enhances slow waves. Sleep 2018; 41(12):zsy176.

97. Zhou J, Liu D, Li X, et al. Pink noise: effect on complexity synchronization of brain activity and sleep consolidation. J Theor Biol 2012;306:68–72.

98. Antony JW, Paller KA. Using oscillating sounds to manipulate sleep spindles. Sleep 2017;40(3): zsw068.

99. Tononi G, Riedner BA, Hulse BK, et al. Enhancing sleep slow waves with natural stimuli. Medicamundi 2010;54(2):82–8.

100. Weigenand A, Mölle M, Werner F, et al. Timing matters: open-loop stimulation does not improve overnight consolidation of word pairs in humans. Eur J Neurosci 2016;44(6):2357–68.

101. Ngo HVV, Martinetz T, Born J, et al. Auditory closed-loop stimulation of the sleep slow oscillation enhances memory. Neuron 2013;78(3): 545–53.

102. Ngo HVV, Claussen JC, Born J, et al. Induction of slow oscillations by rhythmic acoustic stimulation. J Sleep Res 2013;22(1):22–31.

103. Ngo H-VV, Miedema A, Faude I, et al. Driving sleep slow oscillations by auditory closed-loop stimulation–A self-limiting process. J Neurosci 2015; 35(17):6630–8.

104. Leminen MM, Virkkala J, Saure E, et al. Enhanced memory consolidation via automatic sound stimulation during non-REM sleep. Sleep 2017;40(3): zsx003.

105. Besedovsky L, Ngo HVV, Dimitrov S, et al. Auditory closed-loop stimulation of EEG slow oscillations strengthens sleep and signs of its immune-supportive function. Nat Commun 2017;8(1):1984.

106. Debellemaniere E, Chambon S, Pinaud C, et al. Performance of an ambulatory dry-EEG Device for auditory closed-loop stimulation of sleep slow oscillations in the home environment. Front Hum Neurosci 2018;12:88.

107. Garcia-Molina G, Tsoneva T, Jasko J, et al. Closed-loop system to enhance slow-wave activity. J Neural Eng 2018;15(6):066018.

108. Papalambros NA, Weintraub S, Chen T, et al. Acoustic enhancement of sleep slow oscillations in mild cognitive impairment. Ann Clin Transl Neurol 2019;6(7):1191–201.

109. Papalambros NA, Santostasi G, Malkani RG, et al. Acoustic enhancement of sleep slow oscillations and concomitant memory improvement in older adults. Front Hum Neurosci 2017;11:1–14.

110. Ong JL, Lo JC, Chee NIYN, et al. Effects of phase-locked acoustic stimulation during a nap on EEG spectra and declarative memory consolidation. Sleep Med 2016;20:88–97.

111. Grimaldi D, Papalambros NA, Reid KJ, et al. Strengthening sleep-autonomic interaction via acoustic enhancement of slow oscillations. Sleep 2019;42(5):zsz036.

112. Santostasi G, Malkani R, Riedner B, et al. Phase-locked loop for precisely timed acoustic stimulation during sleep. J Neurosci Methods 2016;259: 101–14.

113. Rasch B, Büchel C, Gais S, et al. Odor cues during slow-wave sleep prompt declarative memory consolidation. Science 2007;315(5817):1426–9.

114. Fuentemilla L, Miró J, Ripollés P, et al. Hippocampus-dependent strengthening of targeted memories via reactivation during sleep in humans. Curr Biol 2013;23(18):1769–75.

115. Oudiette D, Paller KA. Upgrading the sleeping brain with targeted memory reactivation. Trends Cogn Sci 2013;17(3):142–9.

116. Rudoy JD, Voss JL, Westerberg CE, et al. Strengthening individual memories by reactivating them during sleep. Science 2009;326(5956): 1079.

117. Oyarzún JP, Morís J, Luque D, et al. Targeted memory reactivation during sleep adaptively promotes the strengthening or weakening of overlapping memories. J Neurosci 2017;37(32):7748–58.

118. Batterink LJ, Creery JD, Paller KA. Phase of spontaneous slow oscillations during sleep influences memory-related processing of auditory cues. J Neurosci 2016;36(4):1401–9.

119. Antony JW, Gobel EW, O'Hare JK, et al. Cued memory reactivation during sleep influences skill learning. Nat Neurosci 2012;15(8):1114–6.

120. Oudiette D, Antony JW, Creery JD, et al. The role of memory reactivation during wakefulness and sleep in determining which memories endure. J Neurosci 2013;33(15):6672–8.

121. Cairney SA, Sobczak JM, Lindsay S, et al. Mechanisms of memory retrieval in slow-wave sleep. Sleep 2017;40(9):zsx114.

122. Honma M, Plass J, Brang D, et al. Sleeping on the rubber-hand illusion: memory reactivation during sleep facilitates multisensory recalibration. Neurosci Conscious 2016;2016(1): niw020.

123. Goldinger SD. Words and voices: episodic traces in spoken word identification and recognition memory. J Exp Psychol Learn Mem Cogn 1996; 22(5):1166–83.

124. Groch S, McMakin D, Guggenbühl P, et al. Memory cueing during sleep modifies the interpretation of ambiguous scenes in adolescents and adults. Dev Cogn Neurosci 2016;17:10–8.

125. Batterink LJ, Paller KA. Sleep-based memory processing facilitates grammatical generalization: evidence from targeted memory reactivation. Brain Lang 2017;167:83–93.

Printed and bound by CPI Group (UK) Ltd, Croydon, CR0 4YY

03/10/2024

01040308-0010